MORE CHOICE

The Canadian Diabetes Microwave Cookbook

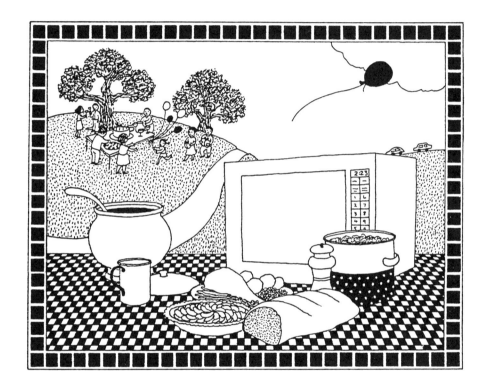

Catha McMaster & Charlotte Empringham

Macmillan of Canada
A Division of Canada Publishing Corporation
Toronto, Ontario, Canada

Canadian Cataloguing in Publication Data

McMaster, Catha, 1958-
 More choice : the Canadian diabetic microwave cookbook

ISBN 0-7715-9432-1

1. Diabetes - Diet therapy - Recipes. 2. Microwave cookery. I. Empringham, Charlotte, 1949-
II. Title.

RC662.M35 1991   641.5'6314   C90-094454-4

1 2 3 4 5 JD 94 93 92 91 90

Design: Avril Orloff
Illustrations: Lindsay Grater
Cover photograph: Jeremy Jones (for recipe see page 140)

Macmillan of Canada
A Division of Canada Publishing Corporation
Toronto, Ontario, Canada

Food Choice Values have been calculated by Christine Bean, R.P.D. (Peterborough Civic Hospital, Weller Street, Peterborough, Ontario), using Guidelines of the Canadian Diabetes Association. This does not constitute an endorsement by the Canadian Diabetes Association.

The endorsement process for this cookbook by the Canadian Diabetes Association is pending.

Recipes were tested in 700-watt turntable microwave ovens.

Printed and bound in Canada by John Deyell Company

ACKNOWLEDGEMENTS

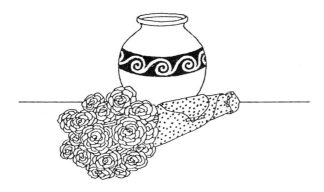

We would like to dedicate this cookbook to our husbands, Jim and Ken, and our children, Jeff and Sara, Michael, Todd, Becky and Ginny. Our loved ones proved to be super taste testers, thorough critics and excellent supporters. Without our families, this cookbook would never have evolved. Thanks to you all!

We also have received wonderful support and information from many others. We would like to thank Heather Beattie, Joanne Brand, Dr. Don Thompson, Dr. Anne Kenshole, Dr. Jim Liston and Eileen Stanbury for reading our manuscript and offering valuable suggestions. We would like to thank Brian O'Connell and Ayesha Hills for compiling the index and Mrs. Christine Bean for checking our food choice values and for her expert information on the Canadian Diabetes Food Choice System.

Without these contributions, we would have encountered much difficulty in seeing this project through to fruition. We deeply appreciate all the input.

FOREWORD

Eating is one of the pleasures of life. For many people cooking is also a pleasure. Just because a member of the family develops diabetes the pleasures of the table and the challenge of producing attractive, tasty and nutritious meals is not diminished, rather it paves the way for new and delicious discoveries. In this book you will find great new ideas for everyday meals and special treats, all based on sound nutritional principles, and easy to follow.

Bon Appetit!

Anne B. Kenshole, M.B.,B.S., F.R.C.P.(C), F.A.C.P.
Internal Medicine, Women's College Hospital
Toronto, Ontario

CONTENTS

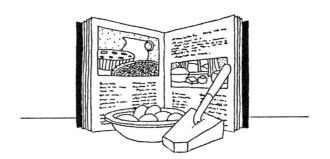

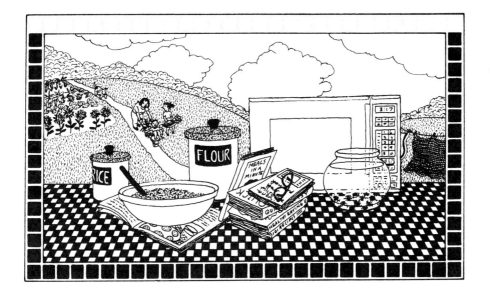

Microwave ovens have been available on the domestic market for about twenty years now. Yet many people are just beginning to learn the techniques needed to successfully cook in a microwave oven. Combination ovens, which combine microwave energy and dry heat, are the recent newcomers to the cooking scene. These ovens have peculiar techniques that cooks would be wise to learn. For a special diet such as the Food Choice System of the Canadian Diabetes Association, a microwave oven is the ideal appliance to use. Your microwave oven allows fast cooking of foods, which will encourage your adherence to your diet. A microwave oven makes clean-up easy by letting you prepare, cook and serve in one utensil. As well, it's easy to clean the oven. The use of a microwave oven instead of a stove reduces your energy consumption 30 to 50%. Add to that savings, the ease of use and the versatility of a microwave oven to boil, steam, poach, simmer, bake, roast and fry. You have the ideal appliance.

This microwave cookbook reflects the diet needs of a person with diabetes. In it you will find an explanation of the Canadian Food Choice Diet and guidelines and microwave cooking tips. More than 150 recipes will show you the way to delicious, healthy meals for every day and special occasions. Yields, calories and per serving exchange breakdown are included for each recipe. The use of convenience foods has been kept to a minimum, eliminating excess salt, additives and hidden sugars. Fresh, wholesome foods are the best way to maintaining optimum health and vitality. Try them prepared in your microwave oven!

MICROWAVE BASICS

In understanding what happens during microwave cooking and why some techniques are used, it is helpful to know what microwave energy is, how it cooks and some of its properties. Take ten minutes and read this section through. It will eliminate some mistakes on the part of a new microwave cook and answer a few questions for the seasoned professional.

MICROWAVE ENERGY

Microwave energy is radio waves that are a little shorter in length than those used by radio stations. Microwave energy can be reflected by metal, can be transmitted through glass and microwave-safe plastics and can be absorbed by food. The radio waves are absorbed by foods to the depth of 2.5 cm (1 in) to 4 cm (1-1/2 in). The radio waves excite the water, fat and sugar molecules in food, causing them to vibrate and rub against each other. This action creates friction, and the resulting heat cooks the food.

Absorption of the microwave energy does not mean there is microwave energy trapped inside the food. After the microwave oven is shut off and its door is opened, the microwave energy dissipates or dies out. Think of your radio. When it is turned off, the song immediately disappears. The same is true of microwave energy in your microwave oven.

The safety of using microwave energy for cooking has been an issue surrounded by confusion. Government and university tests have proven the safety of microwave energy for cooking, and the government has set safety requirements the industry building microwave ovens must follow. There are two categories of energy—ionizing and non-ionizing. Ionizing energy includes X-rays and gamma rays. This type of energy can cause structural changes in cells; these changes pose health risks. Non-ionizing energy includes microwave energy, radio waves and sound waves. It can cause a rise in temperature of cells, but does not interfere with cell structure and therefore poses no health risks.

COVERS: WHAT TO USE AND WHY

Covering the food you place in your microwave oven will do several things. First, it can keep the steam inside the dish to speed cooking. Second, it can prevent splatters. Third, it can absorb excess moisture from food. Determine which of the three purposes the cover should serve, and select a cover accordingly.

Plastic wraps, glass lids, plate (to fit top of bowl), roasting bags:
These covers will hold steam inside a dish, speed the cooking of the food and promote even, thorough heating. Use these covers when cooking vegetables, or tough cuts of meat that need tenderizing, or when reheating and cooking grains and pasta, when moisture retention is important.

Waxed paper:
This cover will prevent splatters and help keep your microwave oven clean. Waxed paper will not hold steam in a dish.

Paper towel:
A paper towel will absorb some moisture or excess fat from food. It can be used to cover cakes that tend to stay too moist on the top or to line baking dishes. Use paper towel to cover roasts and pieces of meat, to prevent splatters.

Foil, terry and linen towels:
This type of cover will act as an insulator and is excellent for aftercooking time. Simply tent food with foil or towel and allow aftercooking time to elapse.

SHIELDING

Shielding is a technique used in microwave cooking to prevent overcooking a portion of food. It is used when cooking a large chicken or turkey or when cooking in a rectangular or square pan. The poultry wings have little meat on them and tend to cook before the rest of the bird. The corners of a square or rectangular pan receive two to three times the exposure to microwave energy as the sides.

To prevent overcooking, place a piece of foil around each poultry wing or lay a 2.5 cm (1 in) strip of foil across the corners of the rectangular or square pan. The foil will reflect microwave energy. Never use more foil than food or arcing (sparks) will occur. Use a fresh piece of foil each time you shield.

PLACEMENT OF FOODS

When cooking more than one food item, such as whole potatoes or an arrangement of hors d'oeuvres, arrange items evenly in a circle on the turntable tray or in the cooking utensil. Even exposure to microwave energy results in even cooking.

Foods should not be stacked or piled.

One food item may be placed anywhere in the oven or in cooking utensil.

STIRRING

Foods can be stirred to rearrange pieces, blend flavors and create smoother puddings and sauces. The door of the microwave oven can be opened any time during the cooking; simply close the door and press "start" to resume the cooking. Forks and whisks provide the best results when stirring sauces and puddings. The fork or whisk tines redistribute smaller clusters of hot food better than a spoon.

REARRANGING AND TURNING FOOD

If the microwave oven does not have a turntable that automatically turns the food, rearrange foods two to three times during the cooking to achieve even cooking. Draw the outer pieces of food towards the centre; move the centre pieces to the edge. Turn casserole dishes a quarter turn two to three times during the cooking.

Large pieces of meat (more than 1.5 kg or 3 pounds) will benefit from being turned over halfway through cooking. Delivery of microwave energy varies from oven to oven, and many ovens tend to have a concentration in one area causing overcooking to occur in this area.

USE OF TURNTABLE

Many microwave ovens have built-in turntables to automatically turn the food for the cook. On a turntable, food will cook 10 to 15% faster. When using a turntable model, cook for the shortest cooking time shown in a recipe. Allow the food to stand. If necessary, return the food to the microwave oven for another minute or two of cooking time.

Turntable ovens offer the added convenience of automatic dish rotation. The food is constantly being rotated through the microwave energy and thus is more evenly cooked.

USING A BROWNING SKILLET

Browning skillets are designed to sear and brown foods in the microwave oven. They should not be used for conventional cooking. The browning skillet has a special bottom that absorbs microwave energy when heated empty in the microwave oven. The bottom of the skillet becomes very hot at 260° to 315° Celsius (500° to 600° Fahrenheit), and the rest of the skillet remains cool. There are ridges or feet on the bottom of the skillet, to protect the floor of your microwave oven and to prevent the conduction of heat from the skillet. Hot browning skillets should not be placed on plastic mats, paper towels or table tops. They should be treated the way you would handle a hot frying pan.

A browning grill has a well around the edge to collect fat and juices. Do not use paper towels or waxed paper with the grill or with the browning skillet, as the heat generated by the dish could set them on fire.

Be sure your microwave oven is clean before using it to heat a browning skillet. Any food on the floor of the microwave oven will bake onto the floor or glass tray. Heat the browning skillet empty, with nothing else in the oven, for a maximum of 8 minutes. (Check the manufacturer's directions for specific times.) Butter, margarine, bacon fat or oil may be added after 1/2 or 2/3 of the preheating time. Non-stick sprays are not recommended for use with the browning skillet, since they will scorch and stain the bottom of the skillet. You will need less butter, margarine, bacon fat or oil than you would use in a frying pan; the amount required depends on the food being seared. Usually you need only to lightly cover the bottom.

POWER LEVEL CHART

POWER	OUTPUT	%	USES
HIGH	700 watts	100%	boil water; brown ground meat; cook fruits and veg; cook fish; cook poultry (under 1.5 kg/3 lb); heat beverages without milk; preheat browner
MEDIUM HIGH	650 watts	90%	heat frozen food without eggs or cheese; heat canned food; reheat leftovers; warm baby food; add milk to scald
MEDIUM	490 watts	70%	bake cakes; cook meats; cook shellfish; cook delicate foods
MEDIUM LOW	360 watts	50%	bake muffins; cook custards; melt butter or chocolate; prepare rice
LOW	200 watts	30%	cook less tender cuts of meat; simmer stews & soups; soften butter & cheese
WARM	70 watts	10%	keep foods warm; rise yeast breads; soften ice cream
DEFROST	245 watts	35%	all thawing
DELAY STAND	0 watts	0%	for aftercooking, start heating later

Note: The above standards chart has been set by the International Microwave Power Institute, an institution governing microwave data throughout the world.

Adapted from *Encyclopedia of Microwave Cooking*, by Madame Benoît, Les Éditions Héritage Inc., 300, Arran, Saint-Lambert, Quebec J4R 1K5

AFTERCOOKING TIME OR STANDING TIME

An important technique to use when cooking or defrosting with microwave energy is called standing time or aftercooking time. This is time in which you allow the food to rest, to let the heat in the outer 2.5 cm (1 in) to 4 cm (1-1/2 in) of food to move to the centre of the food and finish the cooking or defrosting by conduction of heat. It does not matter if the food is in the oven or on the counter for the aftercooking time. However, it is wise to provide an insulating cover for the food, to maintain as much heat as possible. Several covers can be used for aftercooking time. Foil is a good insulator and can be draped over meats and open casseroles. If the cooking utensil has a cover, place a dish towel or quilted placemat over the covered casserole. Food will be slightly undercooked at the start of aftercooking time. Don't worry! It will continue to cook, and will finish perfectly. Allow 30% of the cooking time for aftercooking time to finish dishes beautifully—10 minutes of cooking time = 3 minutes of aftercooking time.

If the aftercooking time is completed and the food requires more cooking, continue to cook on the last power level used for 1 to 2 minutes. Allow another short aftercooking time and check again.

Foods with cooking times of less than 5 minutes do not require aftercooking time.

DIABETIC DIET TIDBITS

- Your diet is *everything* you consume—eat or drink—in a twenty-four-hour period.
- Diabetes does not change the food you need to eat—carbohydrates, proteins, fats and water—to maintain good health. Diabetes does change the way in which the body handles food, and requires a schedule for meals and snacks in order to keep the blood sugar level within the safe range.
- You should always measure your food portions with the same measuring cup and spoon. A kitchen scale is also very useful. After you use these for a period of time, you will be able to estimate accurately.
- Undereating can be just as hazardous as overeating. Be sure to consume all the choices planned for each meal and snack, in order to keep the blood sugar at a safe level until the next meal or snack.
- Plan a snack if there will be more than four hours between meals.
- If a meal is delayed, use some choices from your next meal as a snack. It is best to include a starchy food with a protein food (for example, crackers and cheese). The starchy food will increase the blood sugar level, and the protein food will help to slow down the absorption of the carbohydrates.
- If the evening meal is to be eaten several hours past the normal time, switch the evening meal and the evening snack. Be sure to carry a carbohydrate that is fast absorbing (for example a simple sugar like Life Savers) with you to prevent an insulin reaction in case the snack does not keep the blood sugar level up.

- If you are watching your weight, the following hints are helpful:

  a) Eat only while sitting. This will eliminate nibbling during food preparation time.

  b) To take the edge off your appetite slowly drink 250 mL (1 cup) of water before a meal.

  c) Take your time while eating. Enjoy every bite to the fullest, putting down your fork between bites.

  d) If your meal portions look too small to satisfy on a dinner plate, serve the meal on a salad plate. Your meal will appear larger.

  e) Never have seconds. Make sure you have had your allotment the first time, thus eliminating the need for seconds and possibly overeating.

  f) When the desire to eat arises before a meal is planned, do an enjoyable activity, like knitting or reading for twenty minutes. In that time your desire to eat should pass. A warm drink is often helpful.

  g) When you are successful, do reward yourself, but with a non-edible treat, for example an afternoon doing what pleases you.

  h) Never waste a food choice on a food item you do not really like very much.

THE FOOD CHOICES

The food choice system is a method of measuring food for the diabetic diet to enable flexibility and variety. It also controls the amount of foods containing glucose thereby maintaining as close to normal blood sugar levels. The control of calories aids in maintaining a desirable weight. Choice means a serving of one food can be interchanged with another within the same group. For example: 125 mL (1/2 cup) sliced peaches for 75 mL (1/3 cup) cherries.

There are five food choices or groups of foods: protein, starchy, milk, fruits and vegetables, and fats and oils. Only three of these groups contribute glucose to the blood stream. They are starchy, fruits and vegetables and milk.

Protein

The protein food choices include meat, fish, poultry, cheese and eggs. Your body tissues are made of protein, and you need a certain amount every day to keep the parts of your body in good repair. Any surplus which is consumed is used for energy or stored for future use. Not only are proteins used for building, maintaining and repairing body tissues but they are also used for an important part of hormones and antibodies.

Ideally, meat cuts should look lean with little visible fat marbled throughout the meat.

One Protein Choice contains approximately 7 grams protein and 3 grams fat and will provide approximately 55 calories.

Starchy

The starchy food choices include breads, cereals, cookies, crackers, grains, pastas, rice and vegetables. Starch is a form of carbohydrates referred to as a complex sugar. It does not have the sweet taste of a simple sugar. Approximately 20 minutes after consuming a starch, it is broken down into a simple sugar. This sugar is then able to enter the blood stream. If a person with diabetes has maintained the amount of starch consumed to limited quantities which the insulin can handle, the blood sugar level should remain within a safe range. Be aware of starchy choices that contain hidden fats, such as muffins and cookies.

One Starchy Choice contains approximately 15 g of carbohydrates and 2 g of protein and will provide approximately 68 calories.

Milk

The starch found in a milk choice is lactose, a natural simple sugar. Milk and foods containing milk are excellent sources of calcium, protein and vitamins. People who are allergic to milk may substitute buttermilk, goat's milk, or yogurt. Milk added to cream soups, casseroles or puddings must be included in your selection of choices for the day.

One Milk Choice contains approximately 6 g carbohydrates, 4 g protein, 0 to 4 g fat (depending on the fat content) and will provide 40 to 76 calories (depending on the fat content).

Fruits and Vegetables

The carbohydrate found in fruits and vegetables is a simple sugar, which is absorbed into the blood stream within 5 minutes. Cellulose is a starch which is also found in fruits and vegetables. It is not absorbed into the body but is used as bulk and is necessary to maintain good health. The Fruits and Vegetables Choice also includes dried fruits and juices.

One Fruits and Vegetables Choice contains approximately 10 g of carbohydrates and 1 g of protein and will provide approximately 44 calories.

Vegetables can be eaten when you feel like nibbling. They can be used either raw or cooked and can add interest and fibre to your meal. If these foods are eaten in large quantities, they must be calculated as a Fruits and Vegetables Choice.

Fats and Oils

Fats and oils do not contribute glucose to the blood stream but do provide calories which directly affects your weight. This group includes not only foods such as butter, lard and margarine but also bacon, cheese spreads and nuts.

One Fats and Oils Choice contains approximately 5 g of fat and will provide approximately 45 calories.

Extra

Another food choice referred to as Extra may be used to add interest to your meals. In some cases the amounts must be limited because of the sugar content as well as calories provided. To be calculated as an Extra Choice these foods must contain no more than 2.5 g carbohydrates and provide no more than 15 calories.

Note: Since simple sugars enter the blood stream so quickly, they cause blood sugar level to rise rapidly. Normally the pancreas will automatically release the insulin needed to prevent the blood sugar level from rising too high, thereby allowing the cells to use the sugar. For a person with diabetes, the insulin may not be available when the amount of sugar in the blood is at a high level. This sugar is then spilt over into the urine creating serious consequences. For this reason, it is important to follow the amounts recommended in your diet and to know when your insulin will peak. The person with diabetes must limit the quantity of foods containing simple sugars, but also be sure to obtain sufficient amounts in order to prevent insulin reactions and maintain good health. This is not as difficult to do as it may sound once you understand your diet plan and your insulin requirements.

If you need advice, contact your doctor, a dietitian or talk over your problems with other diabetics. This is when the Canadian Diabetes Association or American Diabetes Association meetings are extremely helpful.

WHAT HAPPENS WHEN FOOD IS CONSUMED?

When the diabetic diet is followed with care and with reference to the Good Health Eating Guide, think of a meal as a time-release capsule, containing the proper choices in the correct amount. A well-balanced capsule would contain starchy food choices and fruits and vegetables food choices which would be the main source of carbohydrates (starches, sugars and cellulose). There must also be protein food choices, milk food choices and fats and oils food choices in order for the capsule to be balanced properly.

When this capsule enters the body, the starches are broken down to simple sugars and enter the blood stream. Simple sugars need not be broken down but are immediately absorbed into the blood stream. Proteins and fats are broken down during digestion and have the effect of slowing down the absorption of the simple sugars into the blood stream. The slower the simple sugars enter the blood stream, the slower the rise in the blood sugar level. Therefore, the balanced time-release capsule will release the sugars at a slow safe rate, preventing a quick rise in the blood sugar level.

Our body uses sugars and fats for energy. Foods which contain carbohydrates turn into sugar or glucose (a simple sugar) in our bodies. The glucose is then carried to all cells of the body and must enter the body cells in order for them to use the sugar for energy. The insulin must be present for this to happen. In the case of the person with diabetes, the insulin is not released when needed but is available at a specific time, according to the type of insulin injected and the time of day it was injected. Different insulins peak at different times. It is important for insulin dependent diabetics to know when their insulin peaks and consume appropriate choices to maintain a safe blood sugar level.

DIETETIC FOODS

Foods that are labelled "dietetic" are not necessarily "diabetic" foods. There are ways of making foods more adaptable for the diabetic diet without spending money on expensive dietetic foods. Remember, anything listed in the ingredients that ends in "ose" is usually a form of sugar. Starch, flour, milk powder, glycerol and dextrin can all cause a rise in the blood sugar level, since they are forms of carbohydrates. In order to maintain good health, treats should be consumed occasionally, including dietetic sweets, which may be allowed.

The following are some examples of how foods can be made adaptable for the diabetic diet without the expense of purchasing a dietetic product.

Whipped Butter

Combine 500 g (1 lb) of butter or margarine with 500 mL (2 cups) skim milk or water. Whip with a mixer or a food processor until thoroughly combined. Use cold ingredients and add the liquid gradually. Makes 2 500 g (1 lb) containers. Store in the coldest part of the refrigerator or freeze.

5 mL (1 tsp) = 1/2 Fats and Oils Choice

Salad Dressing

Combine your favorite salad dressing with equal parts of vinegar. For a change, use wine vinegar. Depending on the kind of dressing used, the choice value will be halved. For example, if French dressing is used, 15 mL (1 tbsp) would be 1/2 Fats and Oils Choice.

Sour Cream

1. Substitute plain yogurt. Try different brands, as they all taste slightly diffcrent.

    125 mL (1/2 cup) = 1 Milk Choice

2. Substitute 125 mL (1/2 cup) cottage cheese whipped with 15 mL (1 tbsp) lemon juice.

    125 mL (1/2 cup) = 2 Protein Choices

Fruit

If you can your own fruit, substitute the syrup with equal parts apple juice and water. Bring the juice and water to a boil and use as you would syrup.

NUTRITIONAL COMPOSITION PER SINGLE CHOICE (FOR MENU PLANNING)				
CHOICE	CARBO	PRO	FAT	CAL
STARCHY	15 g	2 g		68
PROTEIN		7 g	3 g	55
MILK – skim	6 g	4 g		40
2%	6 g	4 g	2 g	58
whole	6 g	4 g	4 g	76
FRUITS AND VEGETABLES	10 g	1 g		44
EXTRA	<3.5 g			<14
FATS AND OILS			5 g	45

Note: 1 Milk Choice can be exchanged for
  1/2 Starchy plus 1/2 Protein
            or
  1/2 Fruits and Vegetables
  plus 1/2 Protein

To receive additional information on nutritional content of foods, contact the Department of Health and Welfare (1-800-387-0700).

CHOICE VALUE CHART
(FOOD COMPOSITION)

ITEM	AMOUNT	FATS AND OILS	FRUITS AND VEG.	STARCHY	PRO	MILK
DAIRY PRODUCTS						
Butter or margarine	5 mL (1 tsp)	1				
	50 mL (1/4 cup)	9				
	25 mL (2 tbsp)	4.5				
	125 mL (1/2 cup)	18				
Cheddar cheese, grated	25 mL (2 tbsp)	1				
	250 mL (1 cup)	3			4	
Cream, half & half	125 mL (1/2 cup)	3				
Cream, sour	250 mL (1 cup)	8				
Cream, whipping	60 mL (4 tbsp)	5				
Milk, evaporated	250 mL (1 cup)					4
Milk	250 mL (1 cup)					2
Egg Yolk	1	1				
Egg White	1					5
Egg, whole dried	25 mL (2 tbsp)				1	
Yogurt, unflavoured	125 mL (1/2 cup)					1
BREADS, CEREALS AND FLOURS						
Bread crumbs	250 mL (1 cup)			4		
Cornmeal, enriched	250 mL (1 cup)			7.5		
Oatmeal	75 mL (1/3 cup)			1		
	250 mL (1 cup)			3.5		
Barley	25 mL (2 tbsp)			1.5		
	250 mL (1 cup)			10.5		
Bulgur	25 mL (2 tbsp)			1.5		
Macaroni	250 mL (1 cup)			5.5		
Noodles	250 mL (1 cup)			4.5	1	
Chow mein noodles	105 g (3-1/2 oz)			4		
Rice	50 mL (1/4 cup)			2.5		
Rice, precooked instant	50 mL (1/4 cup)			1.75		
Spaghetti	50 mL (1/4 cup)			2		
Wheat germ	40 mL (3 tbsp)			1		
Wild rice	50 mL (1/4 cup)			1.5		
Barley flour	250 mL (1 cup)			6		
	15 mL (1 tbsp)			.5		
Rye flour	250 mL (1 cup)			4		
Soy flour	250 mL (1 cup)			1.5	3	
Wheat flour, all-purpose sifted	250 mL (1 cup)			5.5		

ITEM	AMOUNT	FATS AND OILS	FRUITS AND VEG.	STARCHY	PRO	MILK
Cake and pastry wheat flour, sifted	250 mL (1 cup)			5		
Bisquick mix	105 g (3-1/2 oz)	3		4.5		
Cornstarch	50 mL (1/4 cup)			3		

SUGARS AND SYRUPS

ITEM	AMOUNT	FATS AND OILS	FRUITS AND VEG.	STARCHY	PRO	MILK
Sugar						
brown	15 mL (1 tbsp)		1.5			
	125 mL (1/2 cup)		9.5			
	250 mL (1cup)		21			
icing	5 mL (1 tsp)		.5			
	15 mL (1 tbsp		1			
	250 mL (1 cup)		17.5			
white	5 mL (1 tsp)		.5			
	15 mL (1 tbsp)		1			
	125 mL (1/2 cup)		10			
	250 mL (1 cup)		20			
Corn syrup	15 mL (1 tbsp)		1.5			
	125 mL (1/2 cup)		12			
	250 mL (1 cup)		24			
Honey	15 mL (1 tbsp)		1.5			
	125 mL (1/2 cup)		13			
	250 mL (1 cup)		21			
Maple syrup	15 mL (1 tbsp)		1			
Molasses	125 mL (1/2 cup)		10.5			
	75 mL (1/3 cup)		7			
	250 mL (1 cup)		21			
	15 mL (1 tbsp)		1			

FATS AND OILS

ITEM	AMOUNT	FATS AND OILS	FRUITS AND VEG.	STARCHY	PRO	MILK
Chocolate, unsweetened	30 g (1 oz)	3				
Cocoa	50 mL (1/4 cup)	1				
Lard	250 mL (1 cup)	44				
Mayonnaise	15 mL (1 tbsp)	2				
	250 mL (1 cup)	32				
Salad dressing						
blue cheese	15 mL (1 tbsp)	2				
French	15 mL (1 tbsp)	1				
Thousand Island	15 mL (1 tbsp)	1.5				
Olives	105 g (3-1/2 oz)	4				
Vegetable oil	5 mL (1 tsp)	1				
	15 mL (1 tbsp)	3				
	50 mL (1/4 cup)	10				
	125 mL (1/2 cup)	20				
	250 mL (1 cup)	40				

ITEM	AMOUNT	FATS AND OILS	FRUITS AND VEG.	STARCHY	PRO	MILK
MISCELLANEOUS						
Almonds	150 mL (2/3 cup)	9		1	2	
Almond paste	240 g (8 oz)	14		8	1	
Apple, raw, peeled	500 g (1 lb)		5.5			
unpeeled	500 g (1 lb)		6			
Brazil nuts	250 mL (1 cup)	35		2	5	
Cashew nuts	250 mL (1 cup)	7		.5	2	
Chili sauce	15 mL (1 tbsp)		.5			
Coconut, shredded	25 mL (2 tbsp)	1	1			
sweetened	250 mL (1 cup)	5	3			
Currants	250 mL (1 cup)		9			
Dates, pitted	250 mL (1 cup)		13			
Ketchup	15 mL (1 tbsp)		.5			
	50 mL (1/4 cup)		2			
Peanut butter	250 mL (1 cup)	14		3.5	9	
Pecans	250 mL (1 cup)	13		1	1	
Prunes, unsweetened	250 mL (1 cup)		8			
Raisins	25 mL (2 tbsp)		1			
	50 mL (1/4 cup)		2			
	125 mL (1/2 cup)		4			
	250 mL (1 cup)		8			
Walnuts	250 mL (1 cup)	10		1	2	

SUBSTITUTIONS

STAPLES

5 mL (1 tsp)	single-acting baking powder	1 mL (1/4 tsp) baking soda + 2 mL (1/2 tsp) cream of tartar
5 mL (1 tsp)	double-acting baking powder	7 mL (1-1/2 tsp) single-acting baking powder
250 mL (1 cup)	all-purpose flour	250 mL (1 cup) + 3 mL (2 tbsp) pastry flour
250 mL (1 cup)	pastry flour	250 mL (1 cup) less 3 mL (2 tbsp) all-purpose flour
250 mL (1 cup)	self-raising flour	250 mL (1 cup) all-purpose flour + 7 mL (1-1/2 tsp) baking powder + 2 mL (1/2 tsp) salt
15 mL (1 tbsp)	cornstarch, arrowroot or potato starch	25 mL (2 tbsp) all-purpose flour
15 mL (1 tbsp)	all-purpose flour	10 mL (2 tsp) tapioca
250 mL (1 cup)	whole-wheat flour	250 mL (1 cup) all-purpose flour

SEASONINGS

1	medium onion	15 mL (1 tbsp) dried minced onion or 5 mL (1 tsp) onion powder
1	clove garlic	pinch garlic powder or 5 mL (1 tsp) garlic salt; reduce salt in recipe by 2 mL (1/2 tsp)
15 mL (1 tbsp)	fresh herbs	5 mL (1 tsp) crushed dried herbs
15 mL (1 tbsp)	chopped fresh chives	15 mL (1 tbsp) chopped green onion tops
15 mL (1 tbsp)	prepared mustard	5 mL (1 tsp) dry mustard
dash	hot pepper sauce	pinch cayenne or red pepper
30 mL (2 tbsp)	soya sauce	15 mL (1 tbsp) Worcestershire sauce + 10 mL (2 tsp) water
7 mL (1-1/2 tsp)	Worcestershire sauce	15 mL (1 tbsp) soya sauce + dash hot pepper sauce

5 mL (1 tsp)	allspice	2 mL (1/2 tsp) cinnamon + pinch cloves
15 mL (1 tbsp)	chopped fresh ginger	5 mL (1 tsp) ground ginger

CEREALS AND GRAINS

250 mL (1 cup)	fine dry bread crumbs	175 mL (3/4 cup) cracker crumbs
50 mL (1/4 cup)	dry bread crumbs	1 slice bread
125 mL (1/2 cup)	soft bread crumbs	1 slice bread
50 mL (1/4 cup)	dry bread crumbs	175 mL (3/4 cup) rolled oats

DAIRY PRODUCTS

250 mL (1 cup)	butter	250 mL (1 cup) margarine or 225 mL (7/8 cup) shortening + 2 mL (1/2 tsp) salt
250 mL (1 cup)	buttermilk or soured milk	15 mL (1 tbsp) lemon juice or vinegar + whole milk to make 250 mL (1 cup). Let stand 5 minutes. Or 250 mL (1 cup) plain yogurt

MISCELLANEOUS

125 mL (1/2 cup)	raisins	125 mL (1/2 cup) plumped pitted prunes or dates
15 mL (1 tbsp)	active dry yeast	1 pkg active dry yeast or 1 cake compressed yeast
30 g (1 oz)	unsweetened choco-late	45 mL (3 tbsp) cocoa + 15 mL (1 tbsp) shortening, butter or margarine

TOMATO PRODUCTS

325 mL (1 cup)	fresh tomatoes	250 mL (1 cup) canned tomatoes
250 mL (1 cup)	tomato juice	125 mL (1/2 cup) tomato sauce + 125 mL (1/2 cup) water
250 mL (1 cup)	ketchup or chili sauce	250 mL (1 cup) tomato sauce + 50 mL (1/4 cup) sugar + 25 mL (2 tbsp) vinegar

SEASONINGS FOR MEATS AND FISH

Without adding any calories or fat to meat and fish, you can change the flavor in many ways. Herbs and spices contain some oils that help brown meats more efficiently in the microwave oven, and also lend great taste. Some combinations are standards. Try any combination that appeals to you and your family for exciting taste treats.

If you have fresh herbs available, use three times the amount of dried herbs. Fresh herbs have better flavor.

HERBS AND SPICES	ADD TO THESE MEATS AND FISH
Allspice	beef or lamb, ham, pot roast
Basil	chicken, fish, eggs
Bay leaf	beef, lamb, chicken, veal, fish
Caraway	beef, lamb, pork
Celery seed	chicken, pork, beef
Chervil	beef, lamb
Chili powder	beef, pork, eggs
Cinnamon	beef
Cloves	beef, chicken, meat loaf
Coriander	game, pork, sausage
Cumin	chicken, meat loaf, meatballs
Curry	beef, pork, chicken, lamb
Dill	beef, chicken, fish
Fennel	duck, fish, sausage
Garlic	beef, pork, sausage
Ginger	chicken, fish, steak
Marjoram	beef, chicken, fish, sausage
Mint	lamb
Nutmeg	meatballs, eggs
Oregano	beef, chicken, pork, turkey
Parsley	beef, chicken, fish, pork
Rosemary	chicken, lamb, pork, swordfish
Sage	chicken, pork
Savory	beef, fish, pork
Tarragon	beef, chicken, eggs
Thyme	beef, lamb, pork, fish
Turmeric	pork, lamb

EQUIVALENTS

3 tsp	1 tbsp	15 mL
4 tbsp	1/4 cup	50 mL
5-1/3 tbsp	1/3 cup	75 mL
8 tbsp	1/2 cup	125 mL
16 tbsp	1 cup	250 mL
1 oz	2 tbsp	25 mL
8 oz	1 cup	250 mL
16 oz	2 cups	500 mL
32 oz	4 cups	1 L

0.035 oz	1 g
1 oz	30 g
1 pound	500 g
2 pounds	1 kg

1 tsp	5 mL
1/2 tsp	2 mL
1/4 tsp	1 mL
1/8 tsp	0.5 mL
1 tbsp	15 mL
2 tbsp	25 mL

1/4 cup	50 mL
1/3 cup	75 mL
1/2 cup	125 mL
3/4 cup	175 mL
1 cup	250 mL
1-1/2 cups	375 mL
2 cups	500 mL
2-1/2 cups	750 mL

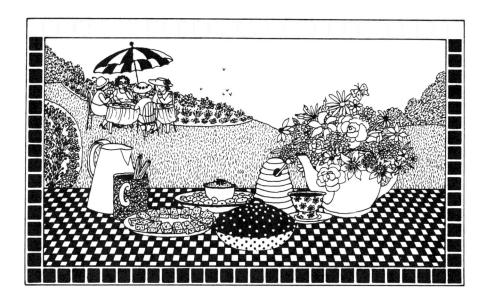

Many exciting beverages can be made with the help of your microwave oven. Remember to count choices from beverages in your daily total. Diet calorie-free sodas, broth made with water and defatted, clear consommé, club soda and mineral waters, and decaffeinated coffee and tea (1 cup per meal) are considered Extra choice beverages. Use as bases for soups, sauces and other drinks without worry. Many beverages can be heated in a microwave-safe glass or mug.

Appetizers offer great nibblers to tide you over to mealtime or to fill in a day's choices. Many can be prepared in advance, even frozen, to be cooked and served as needed. Use spices and herbs freely; they have no choice value. Red and green peppers, spinach and parsley are all Extra foods and act as terrific fillers and garnishes.

Appetizers can be arranged on a microwave-safe plate or serving tray, heated and served. Appetizers should be consistent in size to eliminate uneven heating. Keep appetizers light, and serve only a few to accompany, not overtake, a meal.

QUICK REFERENCE CHART
BEVERAGES AND APPETIZERS

MILK	250 mL (1 cup)	Medium (70%)	2-1/2 to 3-1/2 min.
WATER	250 mL (1 cup)	High	2 to 3 min.
APPETIZERS	4 to 6	High	1 to 1-1/2 min.

TEA

Prepared in a microwave oven, tea will always taste the same—and it is a lot faster than waiting for a kettle to boil and then steeping the tea.

Fill a microwave-safe teapot (one without any metal pieces or trim on it) with cold tap water. Add desired number of tea bags keeping in mind the more tea bags the stronger the tea. The following table gives the times for microwaving at High:

250 mL (1 cup) water	1-1/2 to 2 min.
500 mL (2 cups) water	2-1/2 to 4 min.
1 L (4 cups) water	6 to 8 min.
1.5 L (6 cups) water	8 to 10 min.
2 L (8 cups) water	10 to 12 min.

Be careful not to boil the tea, or it will become bitter. Watch closely the first few times you make the tea and stop the microwave as soon as the water is steaming and small bubbles appear around the edge. Since the flavor will not come out of the tea bags until the water reaches a certain temperature, you can put the teapot in the microwave and program the oven to come on at a set time (if it is equipped with an auto start feature).

Note: The times given above apply also to reheating any beverages.

EACH SERVING   1 Extra Choice

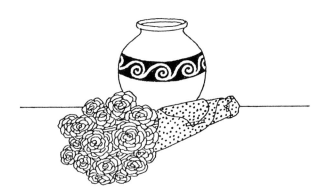

HERB TEAS

Herbal teas don't have to be expensive bag types. Make your own from your spice shelf using a tea ball, strainer or cheesecloth bag. Immerse the herb or spice of your choosing in the boiling water and let it steep. Some herbs and spices take longer to release their flavor. Just be patient; it is worth the wait!

| 250 mL | hot tap water | 1 cup |
| 15 mL | herb, dried or fresh | 1 tbsp |

In a microwave-safe teacup or mug, microwave water at High for 2 to 3 minutes or until water comes to a rolling boil. Remove cup from microwave oven. Place herb in a tea strainer and place in water. Allow to steep 3 to 5 minutes or until desired strength.

HERBS TO TRY:

Dill	Rosemary	Mint	Cinnamon
Whole cloves	Whole ginger	Rosemary	Lemon Grass
Nutmeg	Chicory	Lemon	Thyme
Marjoram	Basil	Coriander	Fennel

FLAVORINGS TO TRY:

Apple peels (washed) and cinnamon
Crushed almonds (use 2 to 3) with shell
Dried apricots, pears, raisins, etc.
 (Count 1 Fruits and Vegetables Choice)
Chamomile flowers
Parsley

Note: Some herb teas contain potent drugs, so be sure to drink a variety of teas rather than only one kind.

| MAKES | 1 serving |
| EACH SERVING | 1 Extra Choice |

FRUIT TEA

Tea can lead the way to many refreshing, easy to prepare and tasty drinks. Put this tea up in a pitcher and keep on hand in the refrigerator all summer long.

1 L	water	4 cups
4	tea bags	4
1/2	lemon, thinly sliced	1/2
1/2	orange, thinly sliced	1/2
1 sprig	fresh mint	1 sprig
	Sweetener to taste (optional)	

In a 2 L (2-quart) casserole, combine water, tea bags, fruit and mint. Microwave at High for 8 to 10 minutes or until water is steaming and small bubbles begin to form. Remove tea bags and fruit. Add sweetener, if desired. Serve hot or cold.

MAKES 4 servings
EACH SERVING 250 mL (1 cup)

1 EXTRA CHOICE

CINNAMON COFFEE

The idea for this distinctive coffee came from my sister-in-law, Pat. She brews coffee in her coffeemaker with a cinnamon stick or dash of cinnamon added. Here is my quick microwave version.

250 mL	hot tap water	1 cup
1	cinnamon stick	1
5 mL	instant coffee	1 tsp

In a microwave-safe mug, combine water and cinnamon stick. Microwave at High for 2 to 3 minutes or until boiling. Stir in instant coffee.

MAKES 1 serving
EACH SERVING 1 Extra Choice

HOT LEMONADE

Hot lemonade is not only wonderfully soothing for a sore throat or cold, but wonderfully warming on any winter day. Or chill it for a summertime refreshment without a choice value.

250 mL	hot tap water	1 cup
	Juice of 1 lemon	
	Sweetener equivalent	
	to 5 mL (1 tsp) sugar	
	(optional)	

In a microwave-safe mug, combine water and lemon juice. Microwave at High for 2 to 3 minutes or until hot. Stir in sweetener, if desired.

| **MAKES** | 1 serving |
| **EACH SERVING** | 1 Extra Choice |

MINT PUNCH

Looking for a pretty punch to serve at festive occasions? This one fits the bill, with its refreshing taste and lovely green color.

500 mL	hot tap water	2 cups
50 mL	dried mint	3 tbsp
500 mL	diet ginger ale	2 cups
	Fresh mint leaves	

Place mint leaves in a teaball, strainer or cheesecloth bag. In a 1 L (1-quart) measure, combine water and mint leaves. Microwave at High for 4 to 6 minutes or until boiling. Steep for 5 minutes. Cool. Add ginger ale. Pour into a punch bowl. Top with mint leaves and serve.

| **MAKES** | 4 servings |
| **EACH SERVING** | 250 mL (1 cup) |

1 EXTRA CHOICE

MULLED CIDER

This taste treat can be made with cider or less expensive apple juice. This recipe lends itself to being increased—simply multiply by the increase (doubling the recipe means 12 to 16 minutes at High and 8 minutes at Medium).

500 mL	apple juice OR cider	2 cups
2	cinnamon sticks, halved	2
4	whole cloves	4
	Sweetener equivalent to 5 mL (1 tsp) sugar	

In a 1 L (l-quart) measure or in 4 mugs, combine apple juice or cider, halved cinnamon sticks and cloves. Microwave at High for 6 to 8 minutes and continue to microwave on Medium (70%) for 4 minutes. Stir in sweetener.

MAKES	6 servings
EACH SERVING	75 mL (1/3 cup)

1 FRUITS AND VEGETABLES CHOICE	10 g carbohydrates
	44 calories

HOT CAROB DRINK

Carob is a flavorful chocolate substitute that contains no sugar. It is a carbohydrate that lends itself to cooking and baking. In most recipes, it can be substituted for cocoa in equal amounts.

15 mL	carob powder	1 tbsp
	Sweetener equivalent to 5 mL (1 tbsp) sugar	
250 mL	skim milk	1 cup
2 mL	vanilla (optional)	1/2 tsp

Combine carob powder and sweetener. In a microwave-safe mug, heat milk at High for 1-1/2 to 2 minutes. Stir in carob powder mix. Add vanilla, if desired.

....

| MAKES | 1 serving |
| EACH SERVING | |

....

2 MILK CHOICES	11 g carbohydrates
	8 g protein
	86 calories

INSTANT CHOCOLATE SYRUP

For the chocolate lover, this is delicious over ice cream or puff pastry shells filled with ice cream or vanilla pudding.

....

175 mL	unsweetened cocoa powder	3/4 cup
pinch	cinnamon	pinch
300 mL	water	1-1/4 cups
5 mL	vanilla	1 tsp
	Sweetener equivalent to	
	125 mL (1/2 cup)	

....

In a 500 mL (2-cup) measure, combine cocoa, cinnamon and water. Stir with a whisk until no dry lumps of cocoa remain. Microwave at High, stirring frequently until mixture comes to a boil, about 2 to 3 minutes. Reduce to Low (30%) and microwave for 5 minutes or until thick and smooth, stirring occasionally. Cool slightly. Stir in vanilla and sweetener. Refrigerate in a covered container for up to 3 weeks.

....

| MAKES | 250 mL (1 cup) |
| EACH SERVING | 15 mL (1 tbsp) |

....

1 EXTRA CHOICE	2 g carbohydrates
	1 g protein
	12 calories

FROTHY HOT CHOCOLATE

The decadent after-ski aperitif!

175 mL	skim milk	3/4 cup
25 mL	Instant Chocolate Syrup	2 tbsp
2 mL	vanilla	1/2 tsp
15 mL	whipped topping	1 tbsp
pinch	cinnamon	pinch

Pour milk into serving mug. Microwave on Medium (70%) for 2 to 3 minutes or until heated through. Add Chocolate Syrup and vanilla and stir briskly. Top with whipped cream and sprinkle with cinnamon.

MAKES	1 serving
EACH SERVING	175 mL (3/4 cup)

2 MILK CHOICES	13 g carbohydrates
	8 g protein
	84 calories

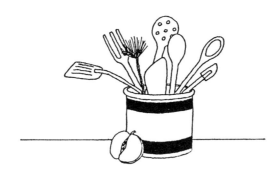

SWISS MOCHA DELIGHT

For a change, try adding a pinch of cinnamon and a couple of drops of peppermint extract.

....

MOCHA MIX

125 mL	instant skim milk powder	1/2 cup
25 mL	unsweetened cocoa powder	2 tbsp
25 mL	instant coffee	2 tbsp

....

Combine all ingredients in a blender or food processor. Blend until well mixed. Store in an airtight jar.

....

To make 1 serving:

25 mL	Mocha Mix	2 tbsp
250 mL	water	1 cup
	sweetener	

....

Place Mocha Mix in a mug and add water. Microwave at High for 2 to 3 minutes or until steam appears. Add sweetener to taste.

   Makes 250 mL (1 cup).

....

EACH SERVING   25 mL (2 tbsp) of mix

....

1 MILK CHOICE   5 g carbohydrates

                                               3 g protein

                                               32 calories

NUTS AND BOLTS

Real party munchies!

1 L	Shreddies	4 cups
500 mL	puffed wheat	2 cups
500 mL	Cheerios	2 cups
500 mL	small thin pretzels	2 cups
250 mL	unsalted peanuts	1 cup
75 mL	vegetable oil	1/3 cup
15 mL	Worcestershire sauce	1 tbsp
5 mL	garlic salt	1 tsp

In a large bowl, mix together Shreddies, puffed wheat, Cheerios, pretzels and peanuts. In a separate bowl, combine oil, Worcestershire sauce and garlic salt. Sprinkle over cereal mixture and toss lightly to coat. Spread a third of the mixture onto microwave-safe pan. Microwave at High for 3 to 5 minutes or until mixtue is hot, stirring after each minute. Spread onto paper towels, in order to absorb excess fat and to cool. Continue with next third of mixture until all mixture has been microwaved.

MAKES	30 servings, 2.75 L (11 cups)
EACH SERVING	75 mL (1/3 cup)

1/2 STARCHY CHOICE	7 g carbohydrates
1 FATS AND OILS CHOICE	3 g fat
	94 calories

SPINACH CREAM SPREAD

This is perfect in sandwiches or as a dip for vegetables or crackers. It stores well in the refrigerator for up to one week.

125 mL	fresh spinach, torn	1/2 cup
125 mL	cream cheese	1/2 cup
125 mL	plain yogurt	1/2 cup
2 mL	salt	1/2 tsp
2 mL	garlic powder	1/2 tsp
2 mL	dried dill	1/2 tsp

In a microwave-safe serving bowl, microwave spinach at High for 1 to 1-1/2 minutes or until wilted. Add cream cheese, mixing well. Continue to microwave at High for 30 seconds to soften cream cheese. Stir in remaining ingredients.

MAKES	6 servings
EACH SERVING	50 mL (1/4 cup)

1-1/2 FATS AND OILS CHOICES	2 g carbohydrates
1/2 MILK CHOICE	2 g protein
	7 g fat
	80 calories

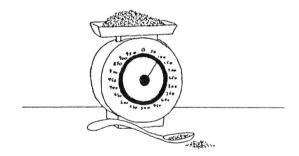

CLAM CREAM CHEESE

Clams come in two basic species—hard-shelled and soft-shelled. The soft-shelled are very high in sodium, so don't eat them too often. The hard-shelled are excellent sources of all B vitamins and are especially suited to cooking.

1	clove garlic, sliced	1
125 mL	cottage cheese	1/2 cup
125 mL	plain yogurt	1/2 cup
5 mL	lemon juice	1 tsp
125 mL	minced clams	1/2 cup
	Freshly ground pepper	

Rub a small bowl with garlic. Place cottage cheese in bowl and heat at Medium (70%) for 30 to 45 seconds to soften. Stir in yogurt, lemon juice and clams. Top with ground pepper. Microwave at Medium (70%) for 30 seconds and serve warm.

MAKES	6 servings
EACH SERVING	50 mL (1/4 cup)

1/2 PROTEIN CHOICE	2 g carbohydrates
1/2 MILK CHOICE	5 g protein
	1 g fat
	42 calories

CHICKEN LIVER PÂTÉ

Liver pâté has long been viewed as an elegant appetizer for entertaining. Serve with toast squares or crackers and garnish with parsley sprigs.

250 g	chicken livers	1/2 lb
1	onion, chopped	1
1	clove garlic, minced	1
125 mL	chicken broth	1/2 cup
50 mL	chopped fresh parsley	1/4 cup

Rinse livers, remove any dark spots and fat, place in a 1 L (1-quart) casserole. Pierce each liver several times. Add onion and garlic clove, mixing gently. Cover with tight lid. Microwave at Medium (70%) for 3 to 5 minutes or until liver is moist but cooked. Mash liver mixture. Stir in broth and parsley. Spoon pâté in a serving dish and garnish with parsley. Serve warm.

MAKES   8 servings

EACH SERVING   50 mL (1/4 cup)

1 PROTEIN CHOICE   3 g carbohydrates

1 EXTRA CHOICE   7 g protein

     3 g fat

     60 calories

SPINACH AND CHEESE STUFFED MUSHROOMS

I have demonstrated these at Canadian Diabetes Association branch meetings, and everyone wanted more!

1 - 300 g pkg	fresh spinach	1 - 10 oz pkg
125 mL	grated Parmesan cheese	1/2 cup
125 mL	grated Cheddar cheese	1/2 cup
125 mL	chopped green onions	1/2 cup
25 mL	parsley	2 tbsp
	Salt to taste	
24	medium mushrooms	24

Wash spinach and drain well. Microwave in a cassserole, uncovered, at High for 4 to 5 minutes. Drain well, pressing extra water out gently. Place spinach in a bowl and add cheeses, onions, parsley and salt. Mix well. (The mixture may be made in advance to this point and refrigerated or frozen. If frozen, defrost before use.)

Remove stems from mushrooms and brush caps. (Do not wash; the mushrooms will absorb water and release it during microwaving, becoming soggy.)

Fill caps with the cheese and spinach mixture and place on microwave-safe cooking utensil. Microwave 12 mushrooms at a time at High for 2 to 3 minutes. Serve hot.

MAKES	8 to 12 servings
EACH SERVING	2 to 3 mushrooms

1 EXTRA CHOICE

COCKTAIL MEATBALLS

The spice of the party!

500 g	lean ground beef OR pork	1 lb
1	egg	1
50 mL	dry bread crumbs	1/4 cup
50 mL	water	1/4 cup
5 mL	beef bouillon concentrate	1 tsp
1 mL	nutmeg	1/4 tsp
1 mL	allspice	1/4 tsp
5 mL	grated lemon rind	1 tsp
15 mL	lemon juice	1 tbsp
	Salt to taste	
25 mL	finely chopped onion	2 tbsp

In a large mixing bowl, combine all ingredients and mix well. Form into 20 small balls using a 5 mL (1 tsp) measure per ball. Arrange half of the meatballs on a microwave-safe rack and cover with waxed paper. Microwave at High for 4 to 5 minutes, rearrange and turn over after 2 minutes. Remove from rack. Repeat with remaining meatballs.

MAKES	20 meatballs
EACH SERVING	4 meatballs

1 PROTEIN CHOICE	2 g carbohydrates
	5 g protein
	3 g fat
	54 calories

OAT BRAN MEATBALLS

Oat bran has recently been hailed as a "wonder food". The fibre it provides is an excellent addition to this recipe and replaces the usual breadcrumbs.

500 g	lean ground beef	1 lb
125 mL	oat bran	1/2 cup
1	egg	1
1	clove garlic, minced	1
2 mL	curry powder	1/2 tsp

Combine all ingredients in a mixing bowl. Form into 2.5 cm (1 in) balls. Arrange 12 in a circle on a microwave-safe dinner plate. Microwave at High for 2-1/2 to 3 minutes. Repeat with remaining meatballs.

MAKES	25 meatballs
EACH SERVING	4 meatballs

3 PROTEIN CHOICES

21 g protein

10 g fat

190 calories

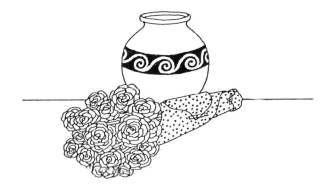

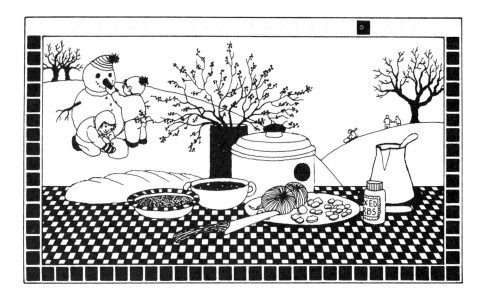

Soups and sauces are wonderfully adaptable to microwave cooking. They can be prepared in large or small quantities, and extra servings can be frozen for future meals. Sauces can be cooked with a minimum of attention—stir once or twice during cooking and at the end of the cooking time. Soups and sauces require cooking time of 2 minutes per 250 mL (1 cup) to boil and 30 seconds to 1 minute to thicken and simmer. Frozen sauces and soups can be defrosted and reheated in one step. Use High power for 3 to 4 minutes per 250 mL (1 cup).

Consommés and stocks make good sense as a staple in a diabetic diet. They make great additions to sauces, can replace gravy and are a base ingredient for hundreds of soups and stews. Both consommés and stocks can be made from scratch or from instant granules and cubes. The advantage to making your own is that you can control the number of additives such as salt, sugar and preservatives.

Soups offer an exciting way for us to use leftover vegetables, rice and pasta, and offer many variations for light dinners and lunches. In this chapter, you will find recipes for consommés and stocks, vegetable soups, cream soups, hearty stews and more.

Sauces provide a wide range of flavors to change everyday fare. They can have a cream, consommé, broth or tomato base. Pour them over pasta, rice, meat and fish to make delicious meals appear magically. Sauces can be frozen and reheated when needed. Avoid freezing milk- or cream-based sauces; they can separate.

Sauces can be prepared and cooked in measuring cups—500 mL (2-cup), 1 L (1-quart) and 2 L (2-quart) sizes are available. Allow room for the sauces to boil. Always stir sauces with a fork or wire whisk for the best distribution of hot and cold. Stir sauce once or twice during the cooking time. Simply open the oven door, stir, shut the door and press the start button. The microwave oven will continue cooking where it left off. Stir sauces at the end of the cooking time to insure a smooth, velvety consistency!

QUICK REFERENCE CHART
SOUPS, STEWS AND SAUCES

FOOD	QUANTITY	POWER LEVEL	TIME
SAUCES	250 mL (1 cup)	High Medium (70%)	2 to 3-1/2 min. to boil 1/2 to 1-1/2 min. to simmer and thicken
SOUPS	500 mL (2 cups)	High High	5 to 7 min. to boil 3 to 4 min. to reheat
FROZEN SOUPS AND SAUCES	250 mL (1 cup)	High	3 to 4 min. to defrost and reheat
STEWS	250 mL (1 cup)	High Medium-Low (30%)	2-1/2 min. to boil 3 min. to simmer

TIPS FOR GRAVIES AND SAUCES

• Blend thickener into cold liquid and stir until smooth.

• If blending into hot liquid, use a whisk or fork to stir.

When using the following thickeners, add the amount indicated to 125 mL (1/2 cup) liquid.

> 10 mL (2 tsp) wheat flour
> 5 mL (1 tsp) cornstarch
> 7 mL (1-1/2 tsp) rice flour
> 5 mL (1 tsp) fine tapioca
> 2 mL (1/2 tsp) potato flour

Add to the following liquids for variations:

> Tomato juice
> Dry white wine and water
> Milk
> Yogurt and water
> Consommé or broth

Remember to account for type of liquid in Choice Values for day.

MUSHROOM SOUP

An ideal appetizer.

250 g	sliced fresh mushrooms	1/2 lb
750 mL	chicken broth	3 cups
10 mL	soya sauce	2 tsp
2 mL	grated lemon peel	1/2 tsp
	Salt to taste	
	Pepper to taste	
10 mL	dry sherry	2 tsp

In a 2 L (2-quart) casserole or soup tureen, combine mushrooms, broth and soya sauce. Microwave at High for 5 to 8 minutes or until boiling. Reduce to Medium Low (50%) and microwave for 5 minutes. Stir in lemon peel, salt and pepper. Microwave at High for 30 to 60 seconds. Stir in sherry and serve.

MAKES	4 servings
EACH SERVING	175 mL (3/4 cup)

1 EXTRA CHOICE	4 g carbohydrates
	17 calories

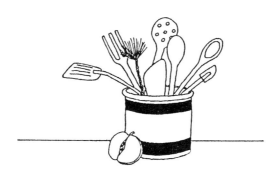

MUSHROOM VEGETABLE SOUP

Add a hearty salad with hard-cooked eggs or cheese and you will have a satisfying meal.

500 g	fresh mushrooms	1 lb
25 mL	margarine	2 tbsp
250 mL	finely chopped carrots	1 cup
250 mL	finely chopped celery	1 cup
250 mL	finely chopped onions	1 cup
1	clove garlic, minced	1
425 mL	condensed beef broth	1-3/4 cups
500 mL	water	2 cups
50 mL	tomato paste	1/4 cup
25 mL	parsley flakes	2 tbsp
1	bay leaf	1
	Salt to taste	
	Pepper to taste	
25 mL	dry sherry	2 tbsp

Brush mushrooms; thinly slice half of them and set aside. Chop remaining mushrooms. In a 2 L (2-quart) casserole, combine mushrooms and 15 mL (1 tbsp) margarine. Microwave, uncovered, at High for 2 to 3 minutes. Add carrots, celery and onions and mix well. Microwave at High for 3 to 4 minutes, stirring once. Stir in garlic, beef broth, water, tomato paste, parsley, bay leaf, salt and pepper. Cover, microwave at High for 5 minutes. Reduce power to Medium (70%) and microwave for 10 to 15 minutes. Purée soup in a blender or food processor. In a small casserole, combine sliced mushrooms in the remaining margarine and microwave at High for 2 minutes. Return puréed soup to large casserole, add sliced mushrooms and sherry. Reheat at High for 3 to 5 minutes.

MAKES	6 servings
EACH SERVING	250 mL (1 cup)

1 STARCHY CHOICE	14 g carbohydrates
1/2 PROTEIN CHOICE	6 g protein
	4 g fat
	124 calories

FRENCH ONION SOUP

A classic favorite, made in much less time than the traditional way.

50 mL	beef bouillon concentrate	1/4 cup
1.25 L	water	5 cups
25 mL	Worcestershire sauce	2 tbsp
500 mL	onions, sliced into rings	2 cups
6	small rounds Melba toast	6
50 mL	grated Parmesan cheese	1/4 cup

In a 2 L (2-quart) casserole or soup tureen, combine bouillon and water and mix well. Stir in Worcestershire sauce and onions. Cover and microwave at High until broth comes to a boil. Reduce power to Medium (70%) and simmer 5 to 8 minutes, until onions are tender. Pour into warmed soup bowls and top with 1 Melba toast round and sprinkle with Parmesan cheese.

MAKES	6 servings
EACH SERVING	250 mL (1 cup)

2 EXTRA CHOICES	6 g carbohydrates
1/2 PROTEIN CHOICE	3 g protein
	1 g fat
	52 calories

TOMATO DILL SOUP

This recipe is perfect for tasting summer any time of the year! Dill and tomatoes combine for a refreshing flavor to liven your palate. Use fresh tomatoes in the summer, canned or frozen tomatoes the rest of the year.

1 L	fresh tomatoes, chopped OR	4 cups
1	can (796 mL / 28 oz) tomatoes	1
125 mL	spaghetti, broken	1/2 cup
15 mL	chicken bouillon powder	1 tbsp
5 mL	salt	1 tsp
5 mL	dried dill	1 tsp

Combine all ingredients in a 2 L (2-quart) casserole. Cover with a tight lid. Microwave at High for 15 to 20 minutes or until boiling. Simmer at Medium Low (50%) for 10 minutes. Allow 5 minutes aftercooking time and serve.

MAKES	4 servings
EACH SERVING	250 mL (1 cup)

2 FRUITS AND VEGETABLES CHOICES	18 g carbohydrates
	3.5 g protein
	.5 g fat
	88 calories

OR

EACH SERVING	125 mL (1/2 cup)

1 FRUITS AND VEGETABLES CHOICE	10 g carbohydrates
	44 calories

CREAM OF TOMATO SOUP

Add baking soda to the milk before combining it with the tomato mixture to prevent curdling.

500 mL	tomatoes, cut in bite-size pieces, juice reserved	2 cups
125 mL	chopped onions	1/2 cup
25 mL	tomato paste	2 tbsp
375 mL	chicken broth	1-1/2 cups
1	bay leaf	1
	Salt to taste	
	Pepper to taste	
150 mL	evaporated 2% milk	2/3 cup
5 mL	baking soda	1 tsp
	Parsley for garnish (optional)	

Place tomatoes and their juice in a 2 L (2-quart) casserole or soup tureen. Add onions, tomato paste, chicken broth, bay leaf, salt and pepper, and mix well. Microwave, uncovered, at High for 5 to 8 minutes or until boiling. Microwave, uncovered, at Low (30%) for 5 minutes. Cool about 15 minutes. Purée in a blender or food processor.

Add milk to the same casserole or tureen and microwave at Medium Low (50%) for 3 to 4 minutes. Do not allow the milk to boil. Add baking soda to the milk, then pour the tomato mixture into the milk. Stir well. Microwave, uncovered, at Medium Low (50%) for 2 to 5 minutes or until hot enough to serve. If desired, garnish with parsley.

MAKES	4 servings
EACH SERVING	175 mL (3/4 cup)

1 FRUITS AND VEGETABLES CHOICE	13 g carbohydrates
1/2 MILK CHOICE	6 g protein
	1 g fat
	85 calories

CREAM OF CELERY SOUP

Milk-based soups need only to be brought to the simmer. If the soup boils, it may curdle.

....

375 mL	chicken broth	1-1/2 cups
125 mL	chopped onions	1/2 cup
375 mL	chopped celery	1-1/2 cups
25 mL	dried parsley	2 tbsp
2 mL	dried basil	1/2 tsp
25 mL	butter	2 tbsp
25 mL	flour	2 tbsp
	Salt to taste	
	Pepper to taste	
250 mL	skim milk	1 cup

....

In a 2 L (2-quart) casserole or soup tureen, combine chicken broth, onions, celery, parsley and basil. Microwave at High for 3 to 4 minutes or until boiling. Reduce power to Medium Low (50%), cover, and microwave 3 to 5 minutes until celery is tender. Place half of mixture in a blender or food processor and blend 30 to 60 seconds or until smooth. Pour into a bowl. Repeat with remaining mixture and set all aside in bowl.

In same casserole or soup tureen, melt butter at High for 30 to 45 seconds. Blend in flour, salt and pepper. Add milk gradually, stirring constantly. Microwave at High for 3 to 4 minutes, stirring every minute until thickened. Stir in vegetable mixture. Microwave at Medium (70%) for 2 to 3 minutes until heated through.

....

| **MAKES** | 4 servings |
| **EACH SERVING** | 175 mL (3/4 cup) |

....

1/2 MILK CHOICE	3 g carbohydrates
1 FATS AND OILS CHOICE	2 g protein
	5 g fat
	71 calories

CREAM OF POTATO SOUP

An Irish favorite.

375 mL	chicken broth	1-1/2 cups
125 mL	chopped onion	1/2 cup
250 mL	sliced potatoes	1 cup
2 mL	dried dillweed	1/2 tsp
25 mL	butter	2 tbsp
25 mL	flour	2 tbsp
	Salt to taste	
	Pepper to taste	
250 mL	skim milk	1 cup

In a 2 L (2-quart) casserole or soup tureen, combine chicken broth, onions, potatoes and dillweed. Microwave at High for 3 to 4 minutes or until boiling. Reduce power to Medium Low (50%), cover, and microwave 3 to 5 minutes until potatoes are tender.

Place half of mixture in a blender or food processor and blend 30 to 60 seconds or until smooth. Pour into a bowl. Repeat with remaining mixture and set all aside in bowl.

Melt butter in same casserole or soup tureen at High for 30 to 45 seconds. Blend in flour, salt and pepper. Add milk gradually, stirring constantly. Microwave at High for 3 to 4 minutes, stirring every minute until thickened. Stir in vegetable mixture. Microwave at Medium (70%) for 2 to 3 minutes until heated through.

MAKES	4 servings
EACH SERVING	175 mL (3/4 cup)

1/2 STARCHY CHOICE	10 g carbohydrates
1/2 MILK CHOICE	3 g protein
1 FATS AND OILS CHOICE	5 g fat
	99 calories

MINESTRONE

Serve this hearty soup with a sprinkle of freshly grated Parmesan cheese on the top and a light salad on the side.

500 g	ground beef	1 lb
250 mL	chopped onion	1 cup
250 mL	chopped celery	1 cup
250 mL	chopped green pepper	1 cup
250 mL	shredded cabbage	1 cup
250 mL	diced potatoes	1 cup
250 mL	sliced carrots	1 cup
1	can (796 mL / 28 oz) stewed tomatoes	1
1 L	water	4 cups
	Salt to taste	
5 mL	Worcestershire sauce	1 tsp
	Pepper to taste	
2	bay leaves	2
125 mL	elbow macaroni, uncooked	1/2 cup
1	can (398 mL / 14 oz) red kidney beans	1

Place meat in a 4 L (4-quart) casserole or soup tureen and break apart. Microwave at High for 5 minutes. Add onions, celery and green pepper, mixing well. Microwave at High for 3 to 5 minutes or until beef is browned. Add cabbage, potatoes, carrots, tomatoes, water, salt, Worcestershire sauce, pepper, bay leaves and macaroni. Stir to combine well. Microwave at High for 8 to 10 minutes or until boiling. Reduce power to Medium Low (50%) and microwave for 15 minutes. Stir in kidney beans and continue microwaving on Medium Low (50%) for 8 to 10 minutes or until macaroni is tender.

MAKES	14 servings
EACH SERVING	250 mL (1 cup)

1 PROTEIN CHOICE	16 g carbohydrates
1 STARCHY CHOICE	10 g protein
	3 g fat
	131 calories

SPLIT PEA SOUP

A hearty, economical soup that can be served for a light meal or with a salad for a full-course meal.

2.5 L	hot water	10 cups
500 mL	dried green split peas	2 cups
750 g	meaty ham bone	1-1/2 lb
	OR	
500 mL	diced ham	2 cups
1	medium onion, chopped	1
	Salt to taste	
	Pepper to taste	
1	bay leaf	1
250 mL	celery cut in 1 cm (1/4-in) slices	1 cup
250 mL	very thinly sliced carrots	1 cup

In a 3 L (3-quart) casserole or soup tureen, combine hot water, split peas, ham bone, onion and seasonings. Cover and microwave at High for 40 minutes, stirring several times. Remove bone; cut off meat and dice. Return meat to the soup with celery and carrots. Stir. Microwave, uncovered, at High for 20 to 30 minutes, or until soup is desired thickness and carrots are tender, stirring occasionally.

MAKES	10 servings
EACH SERVING	250 mL (1 cup)

1 PROTEIN CHOICE	30 g carbohydrates
2 STARCHY CHOICES	12 g protein
	1 g fat
	177 calories

Note: Leftovers will freeze well. Thaw at Defrost and microwave at Medium until heated through. Check manufacturer's directions for quantities and timing.

CLAM CHOWDER

This simple, tasty version of classic chowder has fewer calories than normal. Chowder from scratch contains far less sodium than commercial varieties.

15 mL	margarine	1 tbsp
15 mL	flour	1 tbsp
250 mL	skim milk	1 cup
250 mL	chicken broth	1 cup
250 mL	canned clams	1 cup
2 mL	tarragon	1/2 tsp
2 mL	parsley	1/2 tsp
1 mL	salt	1/4 tsp

In a 2 L (2-quart) casserole, melt margarine at High for 30 to 45 seconds. Stir in flour. Add milk. Microwave at High for 1-1/2 to 2 minutes or until mixture begins to thicken. Stir. Add broth, clams and seasonings. Stir. Continue to cook at High for 4 to 6 minutes or until heated through.

MAKES	6 servings
EACH SERVING	125 mL (1/2 cup)

1 PROTEIN CHOICE	3 g carbohydrates
1 EXTRA CHOICE	6 g protein
	3 g fat
	62 calories

SPAGHETTI SOUP

This soup beats any you can buy in a can and it is so straightforward to make. It's wonderful on a cold, blustery day!

250 mL	dried lima beans	1 cup
750 mL	hot tap water	3 cups
250 mL	frozen corn	1 cup
500 mL	tomato juice	2 cups
250 mL	chicken bouillon	1 cup
120 g	spaghetti, broken	4 oz

In a 3 L (3-quart) casserole, combine lima beans and water. Cover. Microwave at High for 8 to 9 minutes or until boiling. Continue to cook at Medium Low (50%) for 20 minutes. Allow to stand until water is absorbed. Blend in remaining ingredients. Microwave at High for 10 minutes. Reduce power to Low (30%) and simmer for 15 minutes.

MAKES	11 servings
EACH SERVING	175 mL (3/4 cup)

1 STARCHY CHOICE	15 g carbohydrates
	2 g protein
	68 calories

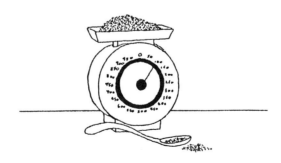

EASY STEW

Quick and easy to prepare.

500 g	stewing beef cut into bite-size pieces	1 lb
1	can (284 mL / 10 oz) tomato soup	1
125 mL	beef broth	1/2 cup
2	medium onions, cut into wedges	2
250 mL	evenly sliced carrots	1 cup
pinch	basil	pinch
15 mL	parsley	1 tbsp
1	bay leaf	1
2 mL	salt	1/2 tsp
pinch	pepper	pinch
175 mL	frozen peas	3/4 cup

In a 3 L (3-quart) casserole, combine all ingredients except peas. Mix well. Cover and microwave at High for 5 minutes. Stir. Microwave at Medium Low (50%) for 60 minutes, stirring 2 to 3 times. Stir in peas. Allow 10 to 15 minute aftercooking time, covered.

MAKES	4 servings
EACH SERVING	175 mL (3/4 cup)

3 PROTEIN CHOICES	22 g carbohydrates
2 FRUITS AND VEGETABLES CHOICES	25 g protein
1/2 FATS AND OILS CHOICE	11 g fat
	287 calories

MICROWAVED OLD-FASHIONED BEEF STEW

That old-fashioned flavor in much less time. Be sure to allow sufficient aftercooking time for maximum tenderness.

50 mL	flour	1/4 cup
5 mL	salt	1 tsp
0.5 mL	pepper	1/8 tsp
1 mL	dry mustard	1/4 tsp
625 g	round steak, 2.5 cm (1-in) thick	1-1/4 lb
500 mL	water	2 cups
5 mL	Worcestershire sauce	1 tsp
500 mL	potatoes, peeled and evenly sliced	2 cups
250 mL	sliced onions	1 cup
250 mL	evenly sliced carrots	1 cup

Combine 25 mL (2 tbsp) of the flour, salt, pepper and dry mustard in a plastic or paper bag and shake well. Trim excess fat from outside of round steak and cut meat into 2.5 cm (1-in) cubes. Shake meat cubes in bag with flour mixture a few at a time.

Place meat in a 3 L (3-quart) casserole and microwave at High for 5 to 8 minutes or until browned, turning 2 or 3 times. Combine remaining flour with water and Worcestershire sauce. Blend until smooth. Pour over meat in casserole and stir to combine. Cover and microwave at High for 5 minutes. Reduce power to Medium Low (50%) and microwave for 25 minutes, stirring 2 or 3 times. Stir in vegetables, cover, and microwave at Medium Low (50%) for 30 minutes. Allow 15 to 20 minutes aftercooking time, covered.

MAKES	4 servings
EACH SERVING	250 mL (1 cup)

1 STARCHY CHOICE	25 g carbohydrates
1 FRUITS AND VEGETABLES CHOICE	26 g protein
3 PROTEIN CHOICES	18 g fat
	365 calories

TOMATO BEEF STEW

The slow cooking is achieved with the Low power level and longer microwave cooking time. Be sure to allow ample aftercooking time for tenderness.

4	medium carrots, cut in 1 cm (1/2 in) slices	4
125 mL	sliced carrots	1/2 cup
500 g	stewing beef cut into bite-sized pieces	1 lb
250 mL	water	1 cup
375 mL	tomato juice	1-1/2 cups
1	medium onion, quartered	1
5 mL	salt	1 tsp
2 ml	garlic salt	1/2 tsp
1 mL	pepper	1/4 tsp
1	bay leaf	1
5 mL	beef bouillon concentrate	1 tsp

Combine all ingredients in a 3 L (3-quart) casserole. Cover and microwave at High for 5 minutes. Reduce power to Low (30%) and microwave for 50 to 60 minutes or until vegetables are tender and beef is fork tender. Allow 10 to 15 minutes aftercooking time, covered. Remove bay leaf and serve.

MAKES	4 servings
EACH SERVING	250 mL (1 cup)

1-1/2 FRUITS AND VEGETABLES CHOICES	15 g carbohydrates
	16 g protein
2 PROTEIN CHOICES	9 g fat
1/2 FATS AND OILS CHOICE	199 calories

MOCK HOLLANDAISE SAUCE

Another sauce with unlimited uses. Pour over vegetables or Eggs Benedict (p. 119) or combine with egg yolks for devilled eggs.

1	egg yolk	1
175 mL	low-fat plain yogurt	3/4 cup
25 mL	lemon juice	2 tbsp
1 mL	salt	1/4 tsp
0.5 mL	dry mustard	1/8 tsp

In a small bowl, lightly beat egg yolk. Add 50 mL (1/4 cup) yogurt, lemon juice, salt and mustard. Microwave at High for 30 to 50 seconds, until thick and smooth. Gradually add remaining yogurt, blending well. If more time is needed to thicken, microwave at High for 20 to 30 seconds.

MAKES   8 servings
EACH SERVING   25 mL (2 tbsp)

1 EXTRA CHOICE

OR

EACH SERVING   50 mL (1/4 cup)

1/2 MILK CHOICE

1/2 FATS AND OILS CHOICE

4 g carbohydrates

3 g protein

2 g fat

48 calories

BASIC WHITE SAUCE

There is no limit to the uses of a basic white sauce, especially when it can be made so quickly and easily in the microwave oven.

250 mL	2% milk	1 cup
15 mL	all-purpose flour	1 tbsp
5 mL	cornstarch	1 tsp
2 mL	salt	1/2 tsp
5 mL	vegetable oil	1 tsp

In a 1 L (1-quart) measure, combine milk, flour, cornstarch and salt. Whisk until completely mixed with no lumps of cornstarch or flour. Microwave at High for 2 to 3 minutes, stirring every minute until mixture comes to a boil and thickens. Stir in oil.

MAKES	4 servings
EACH SERVING	50 mL (1/4 cup)

1 MILK (2%) CHOICE	5 g carbohydrates
	2 g protein
	2 g fat
	46 calories

VARIATIONS

Use Herb Sauce or Béchamel Sauce on cooked vegetables, meat or fish, or as a base for crêpe fillings.

Use Cheese Sauce on cooked vegetables or hard-cooked eggs on toast.

Herb Sauce: To the thickened Basic White Sauce, stir in 2 mL (1/2 tsp) each of dried thyme, basil, oregano and parsley. Values for each serving same as Basic White Sauce.

Béchamel Sauce: Microwave at High for 1 to 2 minutes, 15 mL (1 tbsp) finely chopped onion in the 5 mL of vegetable oil. Stir into thickened Basic White Sauce. Values for each serving same as Basic White Sauce.

Cheese Sauce: Stir 125 mL (1/2 cup) grated Cheddar cheese into thickened Basic White Sauce. Stir until cheese melts. If needed, microwave at High for 15 to 20 seconds to melt cheese. Do not boil, or the sauce may curdle.

MAKES	6 servings
EACH SERVING	50 mL (3 tbsp)

1/2 PROTEIN CHOICE	3 g carbohydrates
1/2 MILK (2%) CHOICE	4 g protein
	4 g fat
	64 calories

MUSHROOM GRAVY

Serve over vegetables or meats for that added pizzazz!

5 mL	vegetable oil	1 tsp
250 mL	chopped mushrooms	1 cup
175 mL	beef broth	3/4 cup
pinch	pepper	pinch
10 mL	flour	2 tsp
5 mL	cornstarch	1 tsp
25 mL	water	2 tbsp

In a 500 mL (2-cup) measure, combine vegetable oil and mushrooms. Microwave at High for 1 to 2 minutes, until mushrooms are heated through. Add broth and pepper, and stir well. Microwave at High for 4 to 5 minutes or until boiling. Reduce power to Medium Low (50%) and microwave for 2 minutes. In a small bowl, blend flour, cornstarch and water to form a smooth paste. Add to mushroom mixture and stir well. Microwave at High for 30 to 60 seconds or until sauce thickens.

MAKES	4 servings
EACH SERVING	50 mL (1/4 cup)

1 EXTRA CHOICE	3 g carbohydrates
	2 g protein
	20 calories

FAT-FREE NO-LUMP GRAVY

So easy, so quick and so good!

250 mL	beef broth	1 cup
10 mL	flour	2 tsp
5 mL	cornstarch	1 tsp
5 mL	ketchup	1 tsp
pinch	salt	pinch
pinch	pepper	pinch
pinch	basil	pinch

In a 500 mL (2-cup) measure, combine beef broth, flour and cornstarch and mix well with a whisk. Stir in remaining ingredients. Microwave at High for 2 to 3 minutes or until gravy thickens.

MAKES	4 servings
EACH SERVING	50 mL (1/4 cup)

1 EXTRA CHOICE	3 g carbohydrates
	1 g protein
	16 calories

SPRINGTIME CHICKEN GRAVY

Gravy without fat is hard to believe but incredible to taste! This gravy can be prepared quickly and used to top sandwiches, meat, potatoes and noodles. Use it often to create new lunches and dinners.

250 mL	chicken bouillon	1 cup
75 mL	plain yogurt	1/3 cup
5 mL	dried mint	1 tsp
2 mL	sage	1/2 tsp
2 mL	thyme	1/2 tsp

In a 1 L (1-quart) measure, heat bouillon at High for 2 to 3 minutes or until it begins to boil. Stir in yogurt, mint, sage and thyme. Microwave at High 30 seconds to 1 minute or until heated thoroughly.

MAKES	6 servings	
EACH SERVING	50 mL (1/4 cup)	

1 EXTRA CHOICE	1 g carbohydrates
	.5 g protein
	.5 g fat
	8 calories

CRANBERRY SAUCE

Cranberry sauce is the traditional partner to turkey dinners. This Cranberry Sauce is more vibrant than its commercial cousins. Fresh cranberries are readily available during the Thanksgiving and Christmas seasons; frozen berries are available the rest of the year.

375 mL	fresh or frozen cranberries	1-1/2 cups
15 mL	lemon juice	1 tbsp
	Sweetener equivalent to	
	175 mL (3/4 cup) sugar	
5 mL	vanilla (optional)	1 tsp

In a 500 mL (2-cup) measure, combine cranberries and lemon juice. Microwave at High for 4 to 6 minutes or until boiling. Stir in sweetener; add vanilla, if desired. Chill until ready to serve.

MAKES	5 servings
EACH SERVING	75 mL (1/3 cup)

1 EXTRA CHOICE	3.3 g carbohydrates
	14 calories

BUTTERMILK MAYONNAISE

This mayonnaise is best made in advance. It requires several hours to set. Anyone trying to reduce and control fat and cholesterol intake will love this version.

2 mL	dry gelatin	1/2 tsp
50 mL	water	1/4 cup
2 mL	dry mustard	1/2 tsp
1 mL	salt	1/4 tsp
250 mL	buttermilk	1 cup
10 mL	chopped green onion	2 tsp
10 mL	chopped parsley	2 tsp

Sprinkle gelatin over 25 mL (2 tbsp) water. Microwave remaining water at High for 10 seconds. Add to gelatin to dissolve. Mix together mustard, salt and buttermilk. Add to gelatin. Stir in green onions and parsley. Chill until mayonnaise begins to thicken. Stir. Chill for several hours before using.

MAKES   325 mL (1-1/2 cups)
EACH SERVING 15 mL (1 tbsp)

1 EXTRA CHOICE

.5 g carbohydrates

.5 g protein

.09 g fat

5 calories

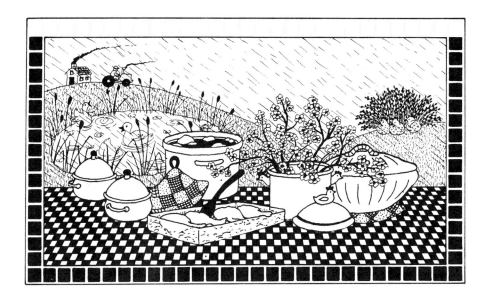

MICROWAVING MEATS
AND POULTRY

In your microwave oven, meats will cook in one-third to one-half the time it takes to cook them in a conventional oven. Since there is no dry heat present, the meat will retain its juices, and its surface will not become dry and crisp. And, for just those reasons, meats cooked in the microwave oven sometimes taste slightly different.

As with the conventional cooking of meats, tender cuts will cook better than less-tender cuts, which require moisture and long, slow cooking in order to soften the tissues. Microwave less-tender cuts of meats at Medium Low (50%) or Medium (70%) to achieve better results. Meat tenderizers and marinades, especially when used overnight, will help to tenderize meats.

Browning occurs when the fat comes to the surface of the meat during cooking and crisps the protein. Time is needed for browning to take place. If meats are cooked in the microwave oven for longer than 10 minutes, browning has a chance to take place.

Meats that are at room temperature before cooking will cook more evenly. Being able to defrost meat in the microwave oven is an important benefit. Not only does meat defrost faster in the microwave oven than it does on its own, but defrosting in the microwave can help to retain the quality of the meat. With the microwave oven, defrosting can be timed so meat will be at its best when it is time to cook it. After defrosting frozen meats, allow a resting time to equalize the temperature in the meat before cooking. All meats should be completely thawed before cooking.

Excellent results can be accomplished when using the barbecue in combination with your microwave oven. Precook meats in the microwave for about 6 minutes per kg (3 minutes per pound), then place on the barbecue to sear the outer surfaces of the meat and produce juicy, tender and flavorful barbecued meats.

Aftercooking is very important when cooking meats in the microwave. Most meats are dense and require this time to allow the temperature to equalize throughout and finish cooking. If the meat is not cooked sufficiently at the end of this time, you can return it to the microwave for additional cooking. As with any food being cooked in the microwave oven, always use the shortest time in the recipe. Meat will become tough if it is overcooked. In some cases, meats will appear done but require aftercooking time to tenderize or improve in flavor. Roasts should be removed from the microwave oven before the desired internal temperature is reached, because they will continue cooking during the aftercooking time.

DEFROSTING MEATS, POULTRY AND FISH

Use of proper techniques for freezing and defrosting will help retain the quality of the meat. Completely unwrap meat to speed up defrosting and to prevent if from starting to cook. Remove plastic or plastic-foam trays— they act as insulators, preventing defrosting from taking place. Also, remove any paper towelling, which will both absorb the juices and attract the microwave energy away from the meat. Elevate the meat on a rack. This will allow the juices to drain away from the meat, thereby preventing the warm juices from cooking the meat. As the meat defrosts, areas that become warm should be covered with foil to shield them from the microwave energy and prevent cooking from taking place.

Time must be allowed for large pieces of meat to thaw completely and to equalize the temperature throughout the meat. Hamburger defrosts very quickly, but should be turned over and around to prevent cooking of the meat in spots. Steaks and chops should be stacked and turned over during defrosting. Six chops or two steaks will defrost in 10 to 14 minutes. (Remember that defrosting is followed by aftercooking or standing time, to allow the temperature of the meat to equalize before starting to cook.) Bacon will defrost enough to separate the slices in 60 seconds for 1 kg (30 seconds for 1 lb) at High power.

Before defrosting whole poultry, always remove the wrappings, or the defrosted juices will heat up and begin to cook the meat they are in contact with. Shield thin spots such as leg tips with foil. Halfway through defrosting time, remove the giblets and neck.

When defrosting fish, remove it from the package and separate if possible; place the fish in the same dish you are going to cook it in. Defrost for half of the time, then rearrange and turn over. Defrost for the remaining time or until fish is defrosted on the outside but still icy in thick areas.

Refer to your microwave oven manual for times per kg/lb for your oven.

MEATLOAF SPECIAL

For a change in taste, substitute ground chicken.

175 mL	dry bread crumbs	3/4 cup
150 mL	tomato juice	2/3 cup
750 g	lean ground beef	1-1/2 lb
125 mL	chopped onions	1/2 cup
5 mL	salt	1 tsp
2 mL	pepper	1/2 tsp
5 mL	Worcestershire sauce	1 tsp
0.5 mL	garlic powder	1/8 tsp

Soak bread crumbs in tomato juice. In a large bowl, combine all ingredients and mix well. Invert a glass juice tumbler in the centre of a 2 L (2-quart) casserole. Surround the glass completely and evenly with meatloaf mix. Microwave at High for 8 to 13 minutes. Allow 5 to 10 minutes aftercooking time. Invert meatloaf onto serving plate and carefully remove the juice glass from the centre (it will contain hot juices). Excellent hot or cold.

MAKES	8 servings
EACH SERVING	1/8 of loaf

3 PROTEIN CHOICES	5 g carbohydrates
1/2 FRUITS AND VEGETABLES CHOICE	22 g protein
	9 g fat
	187 calories

MEATLOAF

For a change in taste, substitute ground chicken.

750 g	ground beef	1-1/2 lb
50 mL	cracker crumbs	1/4 cup
2	eggs	2
125 mL	tomato juice	1/2 cup
50 mL	finely chopped onion	1/4 cup
5 mL	salt	1 tsp
5 mL	Worcestershire sauce	1 tsp
5 mL	garlic salt	1 tsp

Combine all ingredients and mix well. Invert a glass juice tumbler in the centre of a 2 L (2-quart) casserole. Surround the glass completely and evenly with meatloaf mix. Microwave at High for 8 to 13 minutes. Allow 5 to 10 minutes aftercooking time. Invert meatloaf onto serving plate and carefully remove juice glass from the centre (it will contain hot juices). Excellent hot or cold.

MAKES	8 servings
EACH SERVING	1/8 of loaf

3 PROTEIN CHOICES	21 g protein
	9 g fat
	165 calories

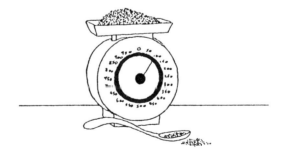

SALISBURY STEAK

625 g	lean ground beef	1-1/4 lb
50 mL	dry bread crumbs	1/4 cup
125 mL	chopped onion	1/2 cup
1	clove garlic, chopped	1
5 mL	prepared mustard	1 tsp
2 mL	salt	1/2 tsp
dash	pepper	dash
1	egg	1
5 mL	vegetable oil	1 tsp
250 mL	chopped mushrooms	1 cup
175 mL	beef broth	3/4 cup
pinch	pepper	pinch
10 mL	flour	2 tsp
5 mL	cornstarch	1 tsp
25 mL	water	2 tbsp

In a large bowl, combine ground beef, bread crumbs, onions, garlic, mustard, salt, pepper and egg. Mix thoroughly. Divide meat mixture into 6 equal portions and shape into patties. Put patties on microwave pan, preferably with a rack. Microwave at High for 7 to 10 minutes, turning once halfway through the cooking time. Allow 5 minutes aftercooking time then check for doneness. If more time is needed to finish cooking, microwave at High for 1 to 2 minutes. Remove patties to serving platter.

In a 500 mL (2-cup) measure, combine vegetable oil and mushrooms. Microwave at High for 1 to 2 minutes, until mushrooms are heated through. Stir in broth and pepper. Microwave at High for 4 to 5 minutes or until boiling. Reduce power to Medium Low (50%) and microwave for 2 minutes. In a small measure, combine flour, cornstarch and water and blend into a smooth paste. Add to mushroom mixture and blend well. Microwave at High for 30 to 60 seconds or until sauce thickens. Serve over patties.

MAKES	6 patties, 250 mL (1 cup) sauce
EACH SERVING	1 patty with 50 mL (1/4 cup) sauce

3 PROTEIN CHOICES	7 g carbohydrates
1/2 STARCHY CHOICE	21 g protein
	9 g fat
	193 calories

CHILI CON CARNE

A favorite on a cold winter night.

500 g	lean ground beef	1 lb
1	large onion, sliced	1
1	green pepper, chopped	1
1	can (540 mL / 19 oz) kidney beans, drained	1
2	cans (540 mL / 19 oz) tomatoes	2
1	can (398 mL / 14 oz) tomato sauce	1
5 to 10 mL	chili powder	1 to 2 tsp
5 mL	salt	1 tsp
1	bay leaf	1
dash	cayenne	dash
dash	paprika	dash

Place ground beef in a plastic colander set in a pie plate. Microwave at High for 3 to 5 minutes, stirring occasionally. In a 2 L (2-quart) casserole, combine beef with onion and green pepper. Mix well. Microwave at High for 2 to 3 minutes, until meat is no longer pink and vegetables are tender. Stir in remaining ingredients. Cover, and microwave at High for 5 minutes. Reduce power to Medium Low (50%) and microwave for 15 to 20 minutes, covered, stirring once or twice.

MAKES	6 servings
EACH SERVING	300 mL (2-1/4 cups)

3 PROTEIN CHOICES	30 g carbohydrates
2 STARCHY CHOICES	25 g protein
	9 g fat
	301 calories

SLIM CHILI

A slimmed-down version of an old favorite.

....

500 g	ground beef	1 lb
1	medium onion, chopped	1
125 mL	chopped celery	1/2 cup
125 mL	chopped green pepper	1/2 cup
5 mL	salt	1 tsp
15 mL	chili powder	1 tbsp
1	bay leaf	1
dash	pepper	dash
1	can (796 mL / 28 oz) tomatoes, undrained	1
1	can 796 mL / 28 oz) kidney beans, undrained	1

....

Place ground beef in a plastic colander set in a pie plate. Microwave at High for 3 to 5 minutes, stirring occasionally. Add onion, celery and green pepper. Microwave at High for 2 to 3 minutes, until vegetables are tender and beef is no longer pink. Spoon beef mixture into a 3 L (3-quart) casserole. Add remaining ingredients and mix thoroughly. Cover and microwave at High for 5 minutes. Reduce power to Medium Low (50%) and microwave for 15 to 20 minutes. Remove bay leaf and serve.

....

MAKES	8 servings
EACH SERVING	250 mL (1 cup)

....

1 STARCHY CHOICE	15 g carbohydrates
2 PROTEIN CHOICES	14 g protein
1 FATS AND OILS CHOICE	9 g fat
	223 calories

SLOPPY JOES

Easy enough for children to make.

250 g	lean ground beef	1/2 lb
50 mL	chopped onion	1/4 cup
50 mL	chopped celery	1/4 cup
250 mL	tomato sauce	1 cup
2 mL	Worcestershire sauce	1/2 tsp
dash	pepper	dash
2	hamburger buns	2

Place ground beef in a plastic colander set in a pie plate. Crumble beef. Microwave at High for 3 to 5 minutes or until almost browned, stirring once. Stir in onions and celery and microwave at High for 2 to 3 minutes or until beef is browned and vegetables are tender.

Transfer meat to a 1 L (1-quart) casserole, crumble, and stir in tomato sauce, Worcestershire sauce and pepper. Microwave at High for 4 to 5 minutes or until bubbling. During 5 minutes of aftercooking time, microwave buns at High for 45 to 60 seconds. Spoon meat mixture over warmed buns.

MAKES	4 servings
EACH SERVING	125 mL (1/2 cup) meat mixture on 1/2 bun

2 PROTEIN CHOICES	20 g carbohydrates
1 STARCHY CHOICE	15 g protein
1 EXTRA CHOICE	5 g fat
	185 calories

SHEPHERD'S PIE

A favorite at our house!

500 mL	peeled, diced potatoes	2 cups
50 mL	water	1/4 cup
25 mL	grated Parmesan cheese	2 tbsp
500 g	lean ground beef	1 lb
250 mL	water	1 cup
15 mL	flour	1 tbsp
10 mL	Worcestershire sauce	2 tsp
5 mL	beef bouillon concentrate	1 tsp
2 mL	celery salt	1/2 tsp
25 mL	chopped onions	2 tbsp
375 mL	frozen peas	1-1/2 cups
125 mL	sliced fresh mushrooms	1/2 cup

Place potatoes in a 2 L (2-quart) casserole with 50 mL (1/4 cup) water. Microwave at High for 8 to 10 minutes, or until potatoes are soft, stirring halfway through the cooking. Allow 4 to 5 minutes aftercooking time. Drain off excess water and mash. Add Parmesan cheese and set aside. Place ground beef in a plastic colander on a pie plate and microwave at High for 3 to 5 minutes, stirring once or twice to separate.

In a 1 L (1-quart) measure, combine 250 mL (1 cup) water, flour, Worcestershire sauce, bouillon concentrate and celery salt. Mix thoroughly. Add onions and microwave at High for 2 to 3 minutes. Add peas and microwave at High for 5 to 6 minutes or until boiling.

In a 1.5 L (1-1/2 quart) casserole, combine vegetable mixture, meat and mushrooms. Microwave at High for 4 to 5 minutes or until heated through, stirring once or twice. Top with mashed potatoes. Microwave at High for 3 to 5 minutes or until potatoes are heated. (If browned topping is desired, bake in 190°C (375°F) oven for 30 minutes until potatoes are lightly browned.)

MAKES	4 servings
EACH SERVING	325 mL (1-1/3 cups)

3 PROTEIN CHOICES	25 g carbohydrates
1 STARCHY CHOICE	26 g protein
1 FRUITS AND VEGETABLES CHOICE	10 g fat
	294 calories

FRENCH CANADIAN TOURTIÈRE

A traditional favorite for Christmas Eve dinner, this dish is a treat any time.

....

PASTRY

250 mL	flour	1 cup
0.5 mL	salt	1/8 tsp
75 mL	lard	1/3 cup
25 to 50 mL	ice water	2 to 3 tbsp

....

FILLING

250 g	lean ground beef	1/2 lb
	AND	
250 g	ground pork	1/2 lb
	OR	
500 g	ground pork	1 lb
50 mL	chopped onion	1/4 cup
1 mL	nutmeg	1/4 tsp
1 mL	cinnamon	1/4 tsp
1 mL	cloves	1/4 tsp
1 mL	salt	1/4 tsp
1 mL	pepper	1/4 tsp
50 mL	beef broth	1/4 cup

....

Preheat conventional oven to 220°C (425°F).

Mix flour and salt. Cut in lard. Sprinkle with ice water and mix lightly. Roll out on lightly floured surface. Line a 22 cm (9-in) pie plate with pastry, reserving enough for a thin top crust. Microwave at Medium (70%) for 3 to 4 minutes.

Place meat in a plastic colander set in a pie plate. Microwave at High for 3 to 5 minutes, stirring occasionally. Blend in onions and seasonings. Microwave at High for 2 to 3 minutes or until onions are tender and meat is no longer pink. Spoon meat mixture into a 2 L (2-quart) casserole. Stir in broth and microwave at High for 1 to 2 minutes.

Fill partially baked pie shell with meat mixture and cover with unbaked top crust. Microwave at Medium (70%) for 10 to 12 minutes. Transfer to preheated conventional oven and bake for 10 to 15 minutes.

....

MAKES   6 servings
EACH SERVING   1/6 wedge

1 STARCHY CHOICE	15 g carbohydrates	
2 PROTEIN CHOICES	16 g protein	
1 FATS AND OILS CHOICE	10 g fat	
	223 calories	

GARDENER'S ZUCCHINI CASSEROLE

Do you garden? Then you already know that one zucchini plant yields dozens of zucchini that you have to cook, pickle, shred, dice, chop, slice, sauté or boil. Here is one more tasty way to serve it up...

500 g	lean ground beef	1 lb
125 mL	chopped onion	1/2 cup
3	small zucchini, sliced	3
125 mL	sliced mushrooms	1/2 cup
500 mL	fresh tomatoes	2 cups
2 mL	garlic powder	1/2 tsp
2 mL	oregano	1/2 tsp
2 mL	basil	1/2 tsp
50 mL	grated Parmesan cheese	1/4 cup

Place ground beef in a 2 L (2-quart) casserole. Microwave at High for 4 to 5 minutes or until beef is browned. Drain off fat. Stir in onions, zucchini, mushrooms, tomatoes, garlic powder, oregano and basil. Cover. Microwave at High for 8 minutes, then Medium (70%) for 10 minutes. Sprinkle with Parmesan cheese. Allow 5 minutes aftercooking time.

MAKES	8 servings
EACH SERVING	200 mL (3/4 cup plus 2 tbsp)

2 PROTEIN CHOICES	5 g carbohydrates	
1/2 FRUITS AND VEGETABLES CHOICE	16 g protein	
	7 g fat	
	146 calories	

MICROWAVED BURGER PIZZA

Serve with a roll and a salad for a complete meal.

500 g	lean ground beef	1 lb
5	saltine crackers, crushed	5
50 mL	finely chopped onion	1/4 cup
50 mL	finely chopped celery	1/4 cup
1	egg	1
5 mL	prepared mustard	1 tsp
5 mL	Worcestershire sauce	1 tsp
1 mL	basil	1/4 tsp
2 mL	oregano	1/2 tsp
125 mL	sliced mushrooms	1/2 cup
30 g	salami, cut into strips	1 oz
1	medium tomato, sliced	1
1/2	green pepper, sliced	1/2
	Pepper to taste	
250 mL	grated Mozzarella cheese	1 cup
15 mL	grated Parmesan cheese	1 tbsp

In a large bowl, mix together well ground beef, cracker crumbs, onions, celery, egg, mustard, Worcestershire sauce, basil and oregano. Pat beef mixture into a 25 cm (10-in) pie plate; form a ridge around the edge. Top with mushrooms, salami, tomato and green pepper. Sprinkle with pepper. Microwave at High for 10 minutes. Top with cheeses. Microwave at High for 1 to 2 minutes or until cheeses melt. Allow 2 to 3 minutes aftercooking time.

MAKES	8 servings
EACH SERVING	1/8 wedge

2 PROTEIN CHOICES	3 g carbohydrates
1/2 FATS AND OILS CHOICE	16 g protein
1 EXTRA CHOICE	9 g fat
	157 calories

PIZZA WITH BEEF CRUST

Friday-night fare.

BOTTOM LAYER

500 g	lean ground beef	1 lb
50 mL	bread crumbs	1/4 cup
1	egg	1
10 mL	onion salt	2 tsp
2 mL	garlic salt	1/2 tsp
1 mL	pepper	1/4 tsp
2 mL	oregano	1/2 tsp
1 mL	basil	1/4 tsp

TOP LAYER

200 mL	tomato sauce	3/4 cup
1 mL	basil	1/4 tsp
250 mL	thinly sliced green pepper	1 cup
125 mL	sliced mushrooms	1/2 cup
125 mL	grated Mozzarella cheese	1/2 cup

Combine ingredients for crust and mix well. Press into a 25 cm (10-in) pie plate and microwave at High for 5 to 8 minutes. Drain off excess fat. Spread tomato sauce over crust and sprinkle with basil. Top with green peppers, mushrooms and cheese. Microwave at High for 5 to 6 minutes or until cheese is melted. Allow 5 minutes aftercooking time.

MAKES	6 servings
EACH SERVING	1/6 wedge

3 PROTEIN CHOICES	10 g carbohydrates
1 FRUITS AND VEGETABLES CHOICE	22 g protein
1 FATS AND OILS CHOICE	13 g fat
	209 calories

PRAIRIE POT ROAST

Great to come home to, especially if your microwave has an auto start feature.

1.75 kg	boneless crossrib chuck OR blade roast	3-1/2 lb
5 mL	dry mustard	1 tsp
2 mL	salt	1/2 tsp
125 mL	chopped onion	1/2 cup
1	can (213 mL / 7-1/2 oz) tomato sauce	1
25 mL	vinegar	2 tbsp
2 mL	thyme	1/2 tsp
1 mL	pepper	1/4 tsp

Trim all fat from roast. Rub dry mustard and salt into the meat. Place in microwave pan. Top with onions.

In a bowl, blend together tomato sauce, vinegar, thyme and pepper; pour over roast. Cover. Microwave at Medium Low (50%) for 40 to 45 minutes for rare, 55 to 60 minutes for medium and 60 to 65 minutes for well done. Allow 15 minutes aftercooking time.

MAKES	10 servings
EACH SERVING	about 90 g (3 oz)

3 PROTEIN CHOICES

2 g carbohydrates

23 g protein

10 g fat

190 calories

GARLIC POT ROAST

Madame Benoît gave this recipe idea to me. The authentic French version includes a topping of butter, margarine or bacon fat; however, this low-fat version gives the original a run for its money.

2	cloves garlic	2
125 mL	water	1/2 cup
1 kg	chuck roast	2 lb
2	bay leaves	2

Peel and cut each garlic clove into 4 slices. Place a saucer upside down in a 2 L (2-quart) casserole. Pour in water. Place roast on top of saucer and lay the garlic slices and bay leaves on the roast. Cover with a tight lid or microwave-safe plastic wrap. Microwave at High for 3 minutes, then at Medium Low (50%) for 25 to 30 minutes. Allow 10 minutes aftercooking time before carving.

MAKES	10 servings
EACH SERVING	90 g (3 oz)

3 PROTEIN CHOICES

21 g protein
9 g fat
165 calories

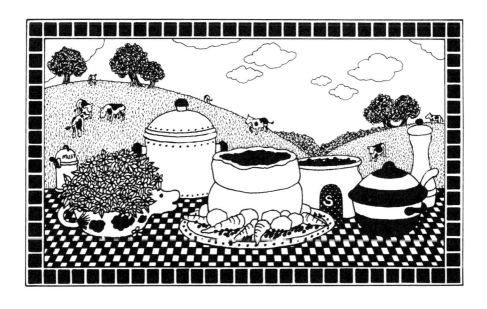

BURGUNDY BEEF

Dinner party fare!

2	slices bacon, chopped	2
500 mL	chopped onions	2 cups
1 kg	stewing beef	2 lb
25 mL	flour	2 tbsp
5 mL	salt	1 tsp
2 mL	thyme	1/2 tsp
1 mL	pepper	1/4 tsp
1 mL	garlic powder	1/4 tsp
175 mL	dry red wine	3/4 cup
175 mL	beef broth	3/4 cup
15 mL	ketchup	1 tbsp
250 g	sliced fresh mushrooms	1/2 lb

Microwave bacon at High for 1 to 2 minutes or until crisp. Set aside. Pour 15 mL (1 tbsp) of resulting bacon fat into a 2 L (2-quart) casserole. Add onions and microwave at High for 2 to 3 minutes or until onions are tender. Remove onions to another dish. Cut beef into 2.5 cm (1-in) cubes, trimming off any excess fat. Add to casserole and microwave at High for 5 to 9 minutes or until browned, stirring occasionally. Add flour, salt, thyme, pepper and garlic powder. Mix well. Microwave at High for 30 seconds. Stir in bacon, wine, beef broth and ketchup. Cover and microwave at High for 5 minutes. Reduce power to Medium Low (50%) and microwave for 30 minutes, stirring occasionally. Add mushrooms and onions. Microwave at Medium (70%) for 5 more minutes. Allow 10 minutes aftercooking time.

MAKES	6 servings
EACH SERVING	125 mL (1/2 cup)

2 PROTEIN CHOICES	8 g carbohydrates
1 EXTRA CHOICE	29 g protein
	12 g fat
	256 calories

BEEF CASSEROLE

Good and hearty.

1 kg	top round steak	2 lb
15 mL	flour	1 tbsp
1	envelope onion soup mix	1
375 mL	water	1-1/2 cups
125 mL	dry red wine	1/2 cup
125 mL	chunks green pepper	1/2 cup
250 g	sliced fresh mushrooms	1/2 lb
1 L	rice	4 cups

Cut steak into 2 cm (1-in) cubes. Dredge in flour by shaking in a paper bag. Combine with onion soup mix, water and wine in a 2 L (2-quart) casserole. Cover. Microwave at High for 5 minutes. Reduce power to Medium Low (50%), and microwave for 12 to 15 minutes, stirring twice. Add green peppers and mushrooms. Microwave 5 to 8 minutes longer on Medium Low (50%). Allow 10 minutes aftercooking time, covered.

MAKES	8 servings
EACH SERVING	125 mL (1/2 cup) rice plus 125 mL (1/2 cup) meat mixture

2-1/2 PROTEIN CHOICES	25 g carbohydrates
1 STARCHY CHOICE	20.5 g protein
1 FRUITS AND VEGETABLES CHOICE	181 calories

FLANK STEAK DINNER

This is a favorite company dish around our house, but my family also loves to have it as a special treat dinner. It is easy enough to serve as an everyday meal.

1 kg	flank steak	2 lb
50 to 125 mL	soya sauce	1/4 to 1/2 cup
25 mL	cornstarch	2 tbsp
25 to 50 mL	dry sherry	2 to 3 tbsp
1	bunch fresh broccoli	1
15 mL	cooking oil	3 tsp
125 mL	chopped onion	1/2 cup
5 mL	salt	1 tsp
500 mL	cooked rice	2 cups

Cut beef across the grain 1 cm (1/4-in) thick and 5 cm (2-in) long. Mix meat with soya sauce, cornstarch and sherry. Cut broccoli into florets. Preheat a large browning skillet at High for 4 minutes. Add 5 mL (1 tsp) of the oil. Add broccoli to skillet, stirring until sizzling stops. Remove broccoli and set aside in a covered casserole. Preheat browning skillet at high for 5 to 6 minutes. Add the remaining oil. Add beef, onions and salt to skillet, stirring until sizzling stops. Cover and microwave at High for 3 to 5 minutes. Add broccoli and microwave at High for 1 to 2 minutes to reheat broccoli. Serve over rice. (See page 124 for instructions on microwaving rice.)

Note: If you do not have a browning skillet, this dish can be made in a casserole. Add 2 to 3 minutes to the cooking time after addition of beef.

MAKES	4 servings
EACH SERVING	175 mL (3/4 cup) meat mixture plus 125 mL (1/2 cup) rice

3 PROTEIN CHOICES	15 g carbohydrates
1 STARCHY CHOICE	21 g protein
1 FATS AND OILS CHOICE	9 g fat
1 EXTRA CHOICE	254 calories

MUSHROOM STEAK

The difference in tenderness is in the aftercooking time. Do not scrimp!

750 g	round steak	1-1/2 lb
1	medium onion, chopped	1
125 mL	sliced fresh mushrooms	1/2 cup
15 mL	parsley	1 tbsp
2 mL	seasoned salt	1/2 tsp
1 mL	pepper	1/4 tsp
1 mL	thyme	1/4 tsp
50 mL	dry red wine	1/4 cup
125 mL	water	1/2 cup

Cut meat into bite-size pieces. Place in a 2 L (2-quart) casserole. Stir in remaining ingredients. Cover and microwave at High for 5 minutes. Reduce power to Medium Low (50%) and microwave for 15 to 20 minutes, stirring occasionally. Allow 10 minutes aftercooking time.

MAKES   6 servings

EACH SERVING   175 mL (3/4 cup)

3 PROTEIN CHOICES   3 g carbohydrates

1 EXTRA CHOICE   20 g protein

                               11 g fat

                               172 calories

SWISS STEAK

A favorite main dish in my cooking classes.

50 mL	flour	1/4 cup
5 mL	salt	1 tsp
1 mL	pepper	1/4 tsp
500 g	round beef steak	1 lb
1/2	envelope onion soup mix	1/2
500 mL	stewed tomatoes	2 cups
50 mL	beef broth	1/4 cup

Combine flour, salt and pepper. Pound meat with a meat mallet to tenderize and flatten until it is 1.5 cm (1/2-in) thick. Cut meat into 4 equal serving pieces and coat with seasoned flour mixture by shaking in a paper bag. Place meat in a 2 L (2-quart) baking dish. Sprinkle with onion soup mix. In a large bowl, combine tomatoes and broth and pour over meat. Cover with microwave-safe plastic wrap. Microwave at High for 5 minutes. Reduce power to Medium Low (50%), and microwave for 10 to 12 minutes. Rearrange meat, recover, and microwave at Medium Low (50%) for a further 10 to 12 minutes. Allow 10 minutes aftercooking time, tightly covered, for meat to become fork tender.

MAKES 4 servings
EACH SERVING 250 mL (1 cup)

3 PROTEIN CHOICES 31 g protein
1 FRUITS AND VEGETABLES CHOICE 10 g fat
209 calories

BARBECUED RIBS

You will not believe how quick and easy these ribs are. The water provides the moist heat needed to tenderize the meat. To prevent the ribs from cooking in too much fat, drain them periodically.

1 kg	meaty spare ribs	2 lb
50 mL	water	1/4 cup
50 mL	soya sauce	1/4 cup
25 mL	vegetable oil	2 tbsp
0.5 mL	cayenne	1/8 tsp
0.5 mL	cinnamon	1/8 tsp
0.5 mL	ground cloves	1/8 tsp

In a 4 L (4-quart) casserole arrange ribs with meat toward the outside edge. Add water. Cover and microwave at High for 5 to 7 minutes. Drain off water. Rearrange the ribs, cover, and microwave at High for 5 to 7 minutes. Drain again, rearrange, and microwave at High for another 5 to 7 minutes. In a small bowl, combine soya sauce, vegetable oil, cayenne, cinnamon and cloves. Mix well. Baste ribs with sauce. Microwave, uncovered, at High for 4 to 5 minutes. Allow 5 minutes aftercooking time.

MAKES	4 servings
EACH SERVING	180 g (6 oz)

3 PROTEIN CHOICES	1.5 g carbohydrates
	22 g protein
	11 g fat
	165 calories

SAUCY PORK CHOPS

Pork must be covered in order to cook evenly and entirely.

4	pork loin chops (500 g / 1 lb)	4
1	can (284 mL / 10 oz) cream of chicken soup	1
50 mL	ketchup	3 tbsp
25 mL	Worcestershire sauce	2 tbsp
2 mL	onion powder	1/2 tsp

Remove fat from chops. Place chops in microwave pan. In a bowl, combine well soup, ketchup, Worcestershire sauce and onion powder. Pour over chops. Cover and microwave at Medium (70%) for 16 to 18 minutes. Allow 5 to 10 minutes aftercooking time.

MAKES	4 servings
EACH SERVING	1 loin chop with 15 mL (1 tbsp) sauce

3 PROTEIN CHOICES	8 g carbohydrates
1/2 STARCHY CHOICE	22 g protein
1 FATS AND OILS CHOICE	14 g fat
	244 calories

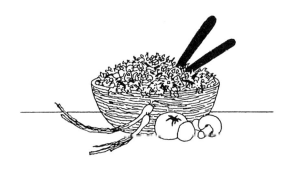

PORK CHOPS IN TOMATO BASIL SAUCE

Covering and aftercooking are important in order to finish cooking evenly and entirely.

4	pork chops	4
250 mL	tomato juice OR V-8 juice	1 cup
5 mL	basil	1 tsp
2 mL	salt	1/2 tsp
1 mL	pepper	1/4 tsp

Trim and discard all fat from chops. Place chops in a pan with thickest portions toward the outside. In a bowl, combine well juice, basil, salt and pepper. Pour over chops evenly. Cover and microwave at Medium Low (50%) for 25 to 30 minutes or until chops are no longer pink. Allow 10 to 15 minutes aftercooking time.

MAKES   4 servings

EACH SERVING   1 pork chop with 15 mL (1 tbsp) sauce

3 PROTEIN CHOICES   2 g carbohydrates

                                        20 g protein

                                        14 g fat

                                        210 calories

MICROWAVED HAM SLICE

A real slice!

1 mL	dry mustard	1/4 tsp
125 mL	unsweetened pineapple juice	1/2 cup
pinch	ground cloves	pinch
500 g	ham slice, 1.5 to 2.5 cm (3/4 to 1-in) thick	1 lb
2 slices	unsweetened pineapple Paprika	2 slices

In a 250 mL (1-cup) measure, blend dry mustard with pineapple juice and cloves. Spread on ham slice. Top with pineapple rings. Microwave at Medium (70%) for 8 to 10 minutes. Sprinkle with paprika. Allow 5 minutes for aftercooking time.

MAKES	4 servings
EACH SERVING	120 g (4 oz) ham slice plus 30 mL (2 tbsp) sauce with 1/2 slice pineapple

3 PROTEIN CHOICES	5 g carbohydrates
1/2 FRUITS AND VEGETABLES CHOICE	21 g protein
	9 g fat
	187 calories

CANADIAN PEAMEAL BACON

The microwave oven offers a perfect way to cook bacon of all kinds, including Canadian or peameal bacon. Peameal bacon won't shrink as much as it does in the conventional oven, and it stays moist.

....

| 500 g | peameal bacon | 1 lb |

....

Arrange bacon on a microwave-safe roasting rack or on an overturned saucer in a larger dish to allow fat to drain away. Cover with paper towel or tea towel. Cook at High for 6 to 8 minutes. Rearranging of pieces may be necessary after 3 minutes cooking time. Allow 3 minutes aftercooking time.

....

MAKES   5 servings
EACH SERVING   90 g (3 oz)

....

3-1/2 PROTEIN CHOICES   26 g protein
1 FATS AND OILS CHOICE   17 g fat
                                    266 calories

GARLIC PORK ROAST

When this roast is cooking, you will be delighted with the aroma that fills the kitchen. Make sure to insert the garlic in the roast. The garlic would be too strong for beef but is perfect for pork!

1.5 kg	pork shoulder roast	3 lbs
2	cloves garlic	2
15 mL	lemon juice	1 tbsp
2 mL	freshly ground pepper	1/2 tsp

Place roast on a microwave-safe roasting rack. Cut garlic cloves in half and insert pieces into slits made in the roast. Rub roast with lemon juice and sprinkle with pepper. If desired, cover with waxed paper or parchment paper. Microwave at High for 2 minutes, then at Medium (70%) for 32 to 36 minutes. Allow 10 minutes aftercooking time.

MAKES	10 servings
EACH SERVING	90 g (3 oz)

3 PROTEIN CHOICES

21 g protein
15 g fat
216 calories

LAMB CURRY

With the addition of a Starchy choice and another Fruits and Vegetables, this dish makes a great meal. The whole family will enjoy lamb prepared in this Middle Eastern way!

500 mL	chopped onions	2 cups
1	clove garlic, minced	1
500 g	lamb, cut into cubes	1 lb
50 mL	flour	3 tbsp
5 mL	curry powder	1 tsp
1 mL	ground ginger	1/4 tsp
5 mL	salt	1 tsp
375 mL	chicken bouillon	1-1/2 cups
500 mL	canned or fresh tomatoes	2 cups
250 mL	chopped apple	1 cup

Place onions, garlic and lamb in a 2 L (2-quart) casserole. Microwave at High for 3 minutes or until lamb begins to brown. Stir in flour, curry powder, ginger and salt. Microwave at High for 1 minute. Add bouillon, tomatoes and apple. Cover and Microwave at High for 8 minutes, then at Medium (70%) for 10 minutes. Stir and serve.

MAKES	6 servings
EACH SERVING	375 mL (1-1/2 cups)

3 PROTEIN CHOICES	11 g carbohydrates
1 FRUITS AND VEGETABLES CHOICE	20 g protein
	8 g fat
	198 calories

ROSEMARY LAMB ROAST

Delicate lamb deserves special treatment. Orange juice and vinegar give the roast a lovely, refreshing flavor and enhance its tenderness.

1.5 kg	lamb shoulder roast	3 lb
15 mL	dried rosemary	1 tbsp
15 mL	orange juice	1 tbsp
15 mL	vinegar	1 tbsp

Place lamb roast on a microwave-safe roasting rack. In a small bowl, combine rosemary, orange juice and vinegar. Rub mixture onto roast. Microwave at Medium (70%) for 30 to 33 minutes. Allow 10 minutes aftercooking time.

MAKES 10 servings

EACH SERVING 90 g (3 oz)

3 PROTEIN CHOICES

21 g protein

15 g fat

216 calories

CRISPY CHICKEN

Yes, you can have crispy chicken out of the microwave oven!

500 mL	dry bread crumbs	2 cups
75 mL	grated Parmesan cheese	1/3 cup
5 mL	oregano	1 tsp
5 mL	basil	1 tsp
2 mL	garlic powder	1/2 tsp
4	chicken pieces	4
	(1 kg / 2 lb)	

Combine the bread crumbs, cheese, oregano, basil and garlic powder, mixing well. Measure out 175 mL (3/4 cup) into a plastic bag. Place chicken pieces into bag and shake to coat. Place chicken pieces in a baking dish with heaviest sections towards the outside of the dish. Cover with waxed paper. Microwave at Medium (70%) for 18 to 20 minutes or until juices run clear. Allow 5 minutes aftercooking time.

Note: The coating mix in this recipe is very easy to prepare and keeps well in the refrigerator. In microwave cooking, natural cheeses (Swiss, Cheddar, Parmesan, Romano) melt, brown and crisp. By using a natural cheese in a coating mix, meat will become brown and crispy.

VARIATIONS

Mexican Crispy Chicken: Substitute chili powder for oregano. Add 0.5 mL (1/8 tsp) cayenne.

Cheddar Crispy Chicken: Substitute grated Cheddar cheese for Parmesan cheese.

MAKES	4 servings
EACH SERVING	1 chicken piece

3 PROTEIN CHOICES	8 g carbohydrates
1/2 STARCHY CHOICE	25 g protein
	10 g fat
	289 calories

HERBED CHICKEN STRIPS

Chicken McMaster is my family's name for this recipe. It is a wonderfully tasty way to prepare chicken for an appetizer or main course. The only appropriate accompaniment is french fries. Prepare them using strips of potato in the same coating and microwave at High for 2 minutes per potato.

250 mL	rolled oats	1 cup
5 mL	basil	1 tsp
5 mL	paprika	1 tsp
2 mL	oregano	1/2 tsp
500 g	boned chicken	1 1b
50 mL	water	1/4 cup
250 mL	tomato sauce	1 cup
125 mL	chopped green onion	1/2 cup

Place rolled oats in a blender or food processor and process for 1 minute or until finely ground. Add basil, paprika and oregano and stir well.

Slice boned chicken into 2.5 by 10 cm (1 by 4 in) strips. Dredge strips in water, then oat mixture. Place strips on a microwave-safe rack. Microwave at High for 4 to 5 minutes or until juices run clear. In a serving dish, combine tomato sauce and green onion for dipping sauce.

MAKES	4 servings
EACH SERVING	90 g (3 oz) chicken

3 PROTEIN CHOICES	4 g carbohydrates
1 EXTRA CHOICE	19 g protein
	8 g fat
	168 calories

SAUCE	50 mL (1/4 cup)
1 EXTRA CHOICE	2 g carbohydrates
	12 calories

CHICKEN PAPRIKA

Hungarian fare with less fat when the chicken skin is removed.

4	equal-sized chicken pieces (1 kg / 2 lb)	4
250 mL	chopped onion	1 cup
10 mL	paprika	2 tsp
2 mL	salt	1/2 tsp
pinch	pepper	pinch
15 mL	flour	1 tbsp
125 mL	skim milk	1/2 cup
75 mL	sour cream	1/3 cup

Remove skin from chicken. Combine onions, paprika, salt and pepper. Place chicken in a microwave pan. Sprinkle with onion mixture. Cover with waxed paper. Microwave at Medium (70%) for 18 to 20 minutes or until juices run clear. Allow 5 minutes aftercooking time.

In a 250 mL (1-cup) measure, combine flour and milk, blending thoroughly. Microwave at High for 1 to 2 minutes or until thickened. Stir in sour cream and combine well. Serve over chicken.

MAKES	4 servings
EACH SERVING	1 chicken piece plus 75 mL (1/3 cup) sauce

3 PROTEIN CHOICES	6 g carbohydrates
1/2 FRUITS AND VEGETABLES CHOICE	23 g protein
1 FATS AND OILS CHOICE	14 g fat
	242 calories

ITALIAN CHICKEN

Removing the chicken skin before cooking reduces the calories.

1	can (398 mL / 14 oz) tomatoes	1
	OR	
500 mL	fresh tomatoes	2 cups
2 mL	oregano	1/2 tsp
2 mL	basil	1/2 tsp
2 mL	salt	1/2 tsp
1 mL	pepper	1/4 tsp
1	clove garlic	1
4	chicken breasts	4
125 mL	grated Mozzarella cheese	1/2 cup
10 mL	parsley	2 tsp

In a large bowl, combine tomatoes, oregano, basil, salt, pepper and garlic. Remove skin from chicken breasts. Place chicken in a microwave pan with thickest sections toward the outside. Pour tomato mixture over chicken breasts and cover with waxed paper. Microwave at High for 18 to 20 minutes. Sprinkle with Mozzarella cheese and parsley. Microwave at High for 2 to 3 minutes or until cheese has melted. Allow 5 minutes aftercooking time.

MAKES	4 servings
EACH SERVING	1 chicken breast plus 175 mL (3/4 cup) sauce

3 PROTEIN CHOICES	5 g carbohydrates
1/2 FRUITS AND VEGETABLES CHOICE	25 g protein
	5 g fat
	211 calories

TERIYAKI CHICKEN

Marinating overnight will enhance the flavor, but this is still yummy when cooked immediately.

125 mL	soya sauce	1/2 cup
1	clove garlic, crushed	1
2 mL	dry mustard	1/2 tsp
5 mL	ground ginger	1 tsp
500 g	boned chicken, thinly sliced	1 lb
5 mL	vegetable oil	1 tsp
4	green onions, chopped	4
50 mL	chopped green pepper	1/4 cup
500 mL	cooked rice	2 cups

In a 1 L (1-quart) measure, combine soya sauce, garlic, mustard and ginger. Add sliced chicken and mix well. Set aside.

In a pie plate, combine vegetable oil, green onions and green peppers. Microwave at High for 2 to 3 minutes, until vegetables are tender. Add chicken, mix well, and microwave, covered, at High for 7 to 9 minutes, stirring once or twice. Allow 10 minutes aftercooking time. Serve over rice. (See page 124 for instructions for microwaving rice.)

MAKES	4 servings
EACH SERVING	250 mL (1 cup)

1 STARCHY CHOICE	15 g carbohydrates
3 PROTEIN CHOICES	23 g protein
1 EXTRA CHOICE	10 g fat
	233 calories

CHICKEN CACCIATORE

A cover of waxed paper will spread the heat out evenly but will not stick like paper towel.

5	chicken pieces	5
1	green pepper, chopped	1
125 mL	sliced fresh mushrooms	1/2 cup
375 mL	tomato juice	1-1/2 cups
2 mL	basil	1/2 tsp
2 mL	oregano	1/2 tsp
0.5 mL	chili powder	1/8 tsp
5 mL	salt	1 tsp
1 mL	pepper	1/4 tsp

Remove skin from chicken pieces. Place chicken pieces in a microwave pan with thickest sections toward the outside. Combine well remaining ingredients. Pour over chicken pieces and cover with waxed paper. Microwave at High for 18 to 20 minutes. Allow 5 minutes aftercooking time.

MAKES 5 servings
EACH SERVING 1 chicken piece plus 75 mL (1/3 cup) sauce

3 PROTEIN CHOICES 5 g carbohydrates
1/2 FRUITS AND VEGETABLES CHOICE 21 g protein
9 g fat
187 calories

CHICKEN KIEV

This classic chicken dish will come out of your microwave oven browned and crisp! The cheese in this recipe will melt, turn brown and become crispy to give perfect results each time.

15 mL	margarine	1 tbsp
1	clove garlic, minced	1
25 mL	lemon juice	2 tbsp
15 mL	chopped fresh parsley	1 tbsp
50 mL	dry bread crumbs	1/4 cup
50 mL	grated Parmesan cheese	1/4 cup
2 mL	paprika	1/2 tsp
500 g	boned chicken breasts	1 lb
1	egg white, beaten	1

Combine well margarine, garlic, lemon juice and parsley. In a small mixing bowl, combine bread crumbs, Parmesan cheese and paprika.

Divide chicken into four pieces. Pound each piece until 0.5 cm (1/4-in) thick. Place 1/4 of the garlic margarine on each piece of chicken. Roll chicken and close securely with a wooden toothpick. Dredge chicken rolls in egg white and then bread crumb mixture. Place chicken rolls on a microwave-safe rack and heat at High for 7 to 8-1/2 minutes. Allow 3 minutes aftercooking time.

MAKES	4 servings
EACH SERVING	1 roll of 90 g (3 oz)

3 PROTEIN CHOICES	3 g carbohydrates
1 EXTRA CHOICE	25 g protein
	14 g fat
	240 calories

CHICKEN À LA KING

An old favorite, with fewer calories when the chicken skin is removed.

25 mL	margarine	2 tbsp
50 mL	flour	1/4 cup
300 mL	chicken broth	1-1/4 cups
250 mL	skim milk	1 cup
0.5 mL	pepper	1/8 tsp
1 mL	paprika	1/4 tsp
2 mL	salt	1/2 tsp
1 mL	onion powder	1/4 tsp
0.5 mL	ground ginger	1/8 tsp
450 mL	diced cooked skinless chicken	1-3/4 cups
250 mL	sliced, fresh mushrooms	1 cup
20 mL	finely diced pimento	1-1/2 tbsp

In a 2 L (2-quart) casserole, melt margarine at High for 30 to 45 seconds. Add flour and blend well. In a large measure, combine chicken broth and milk and microwave at High for 1 minute. Gradually add broth mixture to flour mixture, stirring constantly. Microwave at High for 4 to 5 minutes, stirring after 2 minutes, until thick and smooth. Add pepper, paprika, salt, onion powder and ginger, mixing well. Stir in chicken and mushrooms. Microwave at High for 2 to 3 minutes or until heated through. Add pimento and stir. Cover and allow 5 minutes aftercooking time. Serve over toast, noodles or baking powder biscuits.

MAKES	4 servings
EACH SERVING	150 mL (2/3 cup) sauce with 1 slice toast or 125 mL (1/2 cup) cooked noodles or 1 baking powder biscuit, 5 cm (2 in) diameter.

3 PROTEIN CHOICES	20 g carbohydrates
1 STARCHY CHOICE	24 g protein
1 MILK CHOICE	8 g fat
1 FATS AND OILS CHOICE	290 calories

IF YOU USE BAKING POWDER BISCUITS:	+ 5 g fat
	+ 45 calories

CHICKEN VERONIQUE SALAD

My friends Anne and Paula and I often lunch together with our six youngest children. This recipe was one "guinea pig" I served to them. It serves up elegantly, can be prepared in advance and looks lovely.

500 kg	chicken breasts	1 lb
2	celery stalks, diced	2
125 mL	halved green grapes	1/2 cup
75 mL	plain yogurt	1/3 cup
250 mL	fresh spinach	1 cup
	Parsley to garnish	

Place chicken breasts in a pie plate. Microwave at Medium (70%) for 8 to 10 minutes or until juices run clear. Allow to cool. Remove chicken from bones and cube. In a medium mixing bowl, combine chicken cubes, celery, grapes and yogurt. Serve on bed of spinach leaves and garnish with parsley.

MAKES	5 servings
EACH SERVING	250 mL (1 cup)

3 PROTEIN CHOICES	2 g carbohydrates
1/2 MILK CHOICE	23 g protein
	10 g fat
	190 calories

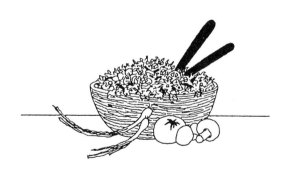

CHICKEN CASSOULET

Chicken and lentils combine to give a hearty meal in one dish. Lentils are one of the legumes that do not require presoaking (the other is split peas), so are fast-cooking additions to many casseroles.

500 mL	cubed cooked chicken, approximately 500 g (1 lb)	2 cups
1	celery stalk, diced	1
1	onion, chopped	1
500 mL	hot tap water	2 cups
500 mL	canned tomatoes	2 cups
250 mL	dried lentils	1 cup
5 mL	celery seed	1 tsp
250 mL	uncooked egg noodles	1 cup

In a 3 L (3-quart) casserole, combine chicken, celery, onion, water, tomatoes, lentils and celery seed. Cover and microwave at High for 20 minutes. Add egg noodles. Cover and continue to cook at Medium (70%) for 20 minutes. Allow 5 minutes aftercooking time.

MAKES	8 servings
EACH SERVING	225 mL (3/4 cup plus 3 tbsp)

3 PROTEIN CHOICES	18 g carbohydrates
1 STARCHY CHOICE	20 g protein
1 EXTRA CHOICE	7 g fat
	228 calories

CHICKEN AND SAUERKRAUT DINNER

I love this meal! The combination of chicken and sauerkraut came from some friends in Lakefield, Ontario. They suggested broiling the chicken, then placing on sauerkraut and topping with cheese. This version incorporates a Starchy choice as well because of the potatoes.

4	potatoes, sliced	4
500 g	boned chicken	1 lb
500 mL	sauerkraut	2 cups
5 mL	caraway seeds	1 tsp
15 mL	prepared mustard	1 tbsp
125 mL	grated Swiss cheese	1/2 cup

In a 3 L (3-quart) casserole, layer sliced potatoes and chicken. Cover. Microwave at Medium (70%) for 8 to 10 minutes or until potatoes begin to soften. In a bowl, combine sauerkraut, caraway and mustard. Spread sauerkraut mixture over chicken pieces. Top with grated Swiss cheese. Cover and microwave at Medium (70%) for 10 to 15 minutes or until juices of chicken run clear. Allow 5 minutes aftercooking time.

MAKES	6 servings
EACH SERVING	90 g (3 oz) chicken plus 175 mL (3/4 cup) vegetable mixture

3 PROTEIN CHOICES	25 g carbohydrates
1 FRUITS AND VEGETABLES CHOICE	24 g protein
1 STARCHY CHOICE	9 g fat
	280 calories

WHOLE ROAST CHICKEN

Does meat brown in the microwave oven? Of course it does. This Whole Roast Chicken browns beautifully with the traditional poultry seasonings. Try the herbal combination for turkey too.

2 kg	roasting chicken (see note)	4-1/2 lbs
5 mL	thyme	1 tsp
5 mL	sage	1 tsp
2 mL	savory	1/2 tsp
2 mL	freshly ground pepper	1/2 tsp

Place chicken on a microwave-safe roasting rack. Combine remaining ingredients in a small bowl. Rub mixture onto bird. Cover bird with waxed paper or parchment paper. Microwave at High for 4 minutes, then at Medium (70%) for 45 to 50 minutes. Allow 15 minutes aftercooking time.

Note: If weight of chicken varies, base cooking time on 26 minutes per kg (12 minutes per lb) at Medium (70%). Allow 10 minutes of aftercooking time as a minimum.

MAKES	6 to 8 servings
EACH SERVING	90 g (3 oz)

3 PROTEIN CHOICES	21 g protein
	15 g fat
	216 calories

BAKED CHICKEN LIVERS

Liver may bring to mind images of shoe leather until you try this tremendous way of preparing it. The liver stays moist and tender and acquires a great taste. Remember to pierce each liver several times with a fork to break the membrane.

500 g	chicken livers	1 lb	
2 mL	thyme	1/2 tsp	
2 mL	sage	1/2 tsp	
2 mL	dry mustard	1/2 tsp	

Rinse chicken livers, remove any dark spots and fat, and pat dry. Pierce each liver several times with a fork. In a 1 L (1-quart) casserole, combine livers with seasonings. Stir. Cover tightly. Microwave at High for 1 minute, then at Medium (70%) for 5 to 6 minutes or until liver is pink. Allow 5 minutes aftercooking time.

MAKES   5 servings
EACH SERVING   90 g (3 oz)

3 PROTEIN CHOICES   3 g carbohydrates
1/2 MILK CHOICE   26 g protein
                                         4 g fat
                                         164 calories

TURKEY TETRAZZINI

A great way to use up those turkey leftovers.

15 mL	margarine	1 tbsp
75 mL	flour	1/3 cup
625 mL	chicken broth	2-1/2 cups
250 mL	skim milk	1 cup
50 mL	dry sherry	1/4 cup
10 mL	parsley	2 tsp
5 mL	salt	1 tsp
2 mL	nutmeg	1/2 tsp
2 mL	onion powder	1/2 tsp
pinch	pepper	pinch
pinch	paprika	pinch
250 g	thin noodles	1/2 lb
125 mL	sliced, fresh mushrooms	1/2 cup
1 L	chopped cooked turkey	4 cups
50 mL	grated Parmesan cheese	1/4 cup

In a large measure, melt margarine at High for 30 to 45 seconds. Blend in flour until smooth. Add broth and milk and whisk to eliminate lumps. Microwave at High for 6 to 8 minutes or until boiling, stirring halfway through cooking time. Add sherry, parsley, salt, nutmeg, onion powder, pepper and paprika. Microwave at High for 1 to 2 minutes or until thickened. Set aside.

In a large casserole, combine noodles with enough water to cover and "swim." Microwave at High for 6 minutes; reduce power to Medium (70%) for 6 minutes. Allow to aftercook for 5 minutes, then drain.

Meanwhile, reheat the sauce at High for 1 to 2 minutes. Add mushrooms. Combine sauce, noodles and turkey in a 3 L (3-quart) casserole. Cover and microwave at Medium (70%) for 8 to 10 minutes or until heated through. Top with Parmesan cheese. Allow 5 to 8 minutes aftercooking time.

MAKES	8 servings
EACH SERVING	250 mL (1 cup)

3 PROTEIN CHOICES	30 g carbohydrates
2 STARCHY CHOICES	23 g protein
	11 g fat
	311 calories

TURKEY SAUSAGE PATTIES

I get discouraged whenever I read the bacon and sausage packages at the grocery store—they contain so many chemicals! This recipe is easy to prepare and tasty, and it uses up leftovers. What more could you ask for?

500 g	cooked turkey	1 lb
50 mL	dry bread crumbs	1/4 cup
1 mL	pepper	1/4 tsp
1 mL	ground ginger	1/4 tsp
1 mL	ground sage	1/4 tsp

Grind cooked turkey in food processor or blender. Combine ground turkey with bread crumbs and seasonings. Form into 8 patties. Arrange patties on a microwave-safe dinner plate. Microwave at High for 2 to 3 minutes. Serve immediately.

MAKES	8 patties
EACH SERVING	1 patty

2 PROTEIN CHOICES

14 g protein

6 g fat

118 calories

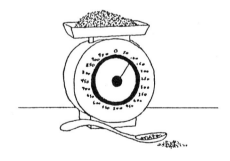

BROWN RICE AND SHRIMP CASSEROLE

This is a quick and easy dish to prepare and serves up beautifully on a buffet or dinner table. The combination of vegetables, shrimp and rice seasoned with cinnamon and nutmeg is very pleasing to the palate.

15 mL	oil OR margarine	1 tbsp
250 mL	uncooked brown rice	1 cup
500 mL	chicken broth	2 cups
250 g	uncooked shrimp	1/2 lb
500 mL	canned tomatoes	2 cups
2	carrots, sliced	2
2	potatoes, cubed	2
1 mL	cinnamon	1/4 tsp
2 mL	nutmeg	1/2 tsp
1	clove garlic, minced	1

In a 3 L (3-quart) casserole, microwave oil or margarine at High for 30 to 45 seconds or until hot. Stir in rice until well coated. Microwave at High for 1-1/2 to 2 minutes or until rice begins to sizzle. Add broth. Cover dish. Microwave at High for 4 to 5 minutes, then at Medium Low (50%) for 10 to 15 minutes or until rice is tender. Allow 5 minutes aftercooking time.

Peel and devein shrimp. Add shrimp and remaining ingredients to rice. Cover. Microwave at High for 5 minutes, then continue to cook at Low (30%) for 30 to 45 minutes or until vegetables are tender.

MAKES	4 servings
EACH SERVING	300 mL (1-1/4 cups)

2 FRUITS AND VEGETABLES CHOICES	33 g carbohydrates
1 STARCHY CHOICE	8 g protein
1/2 MILK CHOICE	2.6 g fat
	188 calories

POACHED FISH

Quick and easy!

500 g	fish fillets	1 lb
	Salt to taste	
	Pepper to taste	
1 mL	ground bay leaf	1/4 tsp
1	medium onion, chopped	1
2	slices lemon	2
	Parsley as garnish	

Place fish fillets in a microwave pan. Sprinkle with salt, pepper and ground bay leaf. Top with onion and lemon slices. Cover with waxed paper and microwave at High for 4 to 6 minutes. Allow 3 to 4 minutes aftercooking time. Check for doneness. Microwave an extra minute if necessary. Sprinkle with parsley before serving.

MAKES 4 servings
EACH SERVING about 90 g (3 oz)

3 PROTEIN CHOICES

1 g carbohydrates

21 g protein

9 g fat

165 calories

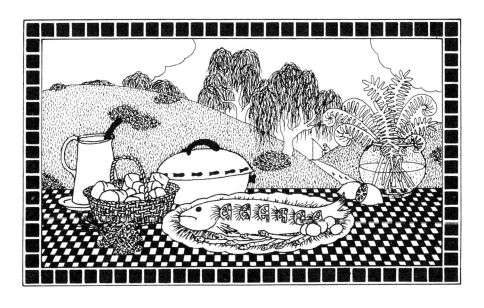

BAKED PERCH

This dish makes dinnertime the easiest time of day. Cook rice and make a vegetable salad for a complete meal.

500 g	perch fillets	1 lb
1 mL	freshly ground pepper	1/4 tsp
1 mL	garlic powder	1/4 tsp
50 mL	sliced mushrooms	1/4 cup
1	red pepper, sliced	1

Arrange perch fillets in square baking dish. Sprinkle with pepper and garlic powder. Arrange mushrooms and red peppers on top of fillets. Cover. Microwave at High for 5 to 6 minutes or until thickest part of fish just turns opaque.

MAKES	5 servings
EACH SERVING	90 g (3 oz)

3 PROTEIN CHOICES	2 g carbohydrates
1/2 EXTRA CHOICE	22 g protein
	10 g fat
	189 calories

CREOLE FISH

A colorful, tantalizing dish!

500 g	fish fillets	1 lb
25 mL	finely chopped green pepper	2 tbsp
1	small onion, chopped	1
50 mL	chopped celery	1/4 cup
2 mL	salt	1/2 tsp
1 mL	oregano	1/4 tsp
0.5 mL	pepper	1/8 tsp
250 mL	stewed tomatoes	1 cup
250 mL	frozen corn, thawed to separate	1 cup

Place fish fillets in a microwave pan, cover, and microwave at Medium (70%) for 5 to 7 minutes. Combine remaining ingredients and mix well. Spoon over fish. Cover and microwave at High for 5 to 8 minutes or until heated through. Allow 5 minutes aftercooking time.

MAKES 4 servings

EACH SERVING 1/4 of fish fillets plus 125 mL (1/2 cup) sauce

3 PROTEIN CHOICES

1 FRUITS AND VEGETABLES CHOICE

12 g carbohydrates

23 g protein

233 calories

LEMON LIME SALMON

I found this recipe in Nova Scotia during a trip for Panasonic. The host distributor served it during a dealer presentation. What a hit!

2 mL	lemon zest	1/2 tsp
2 mL	lime zest	1/2 tsp
15 mL	margarine	1 tbsp
500-g	salmon fillet	1-lb

In a small bowl, stir the lemon and lime zests into the margarine. Microwave at High for 30 to 45 seconds, or until margarine is melted. Brush onto salmon fillet. (If time allows, refrigerate for 1 hour before cooking.)

Microwave salmon at High for 4 to 5 minutes. Allow 3 minutes aftercooking time.

MAKES	4 servings
EACH SERVING	90 g (3 oz)

3 PROTEIN CHOICES

22 g protein

12 g fat

197 calories

SALMON RING

Well worth the effort!

375 mL	water	1-1/2 cups
125 mL	uncooked long grain rice	1/2 cup
5 mL	butter OR margarine	1 tsp
250 mL	finely chopped celery	1 cup
50 mL	finely chopped onion	1/4 cup
2	eggs	2
dash	pepper	dash
1	can (220 g / 7-3/4 oz) salmon, with juices	1
125 mL	skim milk	1/2 cup
dash	cinnamon	dash
dash	nutmeg	dash
dash	allspice	dash
125 mL	grated Swiss cheese	1/2 cup

Combine water and rice in a 3 L (3-quart) casserole. Microwave at High for 6 to 8 minutes or until boiling. Reduce power to Medium (70%) and microwave for 8 to 10 minutes or until all water is absorbed.

In a small casserole, melt butter or margarine at High for 30 to 45 seconds. Add celery and onions, mixing well. Microwave at High for 3 to 4 minutes or until vegetables are tender.

Combine 1 egg and pepper with rice. Press into the bottom of a ring mould or around a glass juice tumbler in the centre of a pie plate.

Combine vegetables, salmon, 1 egg, milk, cinnamon, nutmeg, allspice and half the cheese. Spread over rice mixture. Microwave at Medium Low (50%) for 8 to 12 minutes. Top with remaining cheese. Allow 5 to 8 minutes aftercooking time. When done, a toothpick inserted in the centre should come out clean. If more cooking time is needed, microwave at Medium Low (50%) for 30-second intervals.

MAKES	6 servings
EACH SERVING	175 mL (3/4 cup)

2 PROTEIN CHOICES	15 g carbohydrates
1 STARCHY CHOICE	15 g protein
	6 g fat
	178 calories

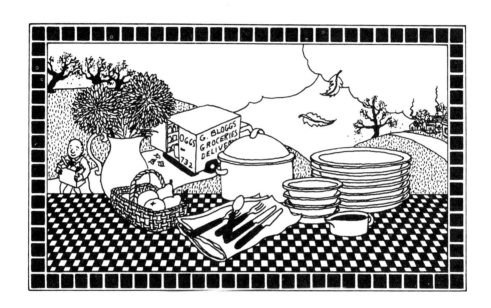

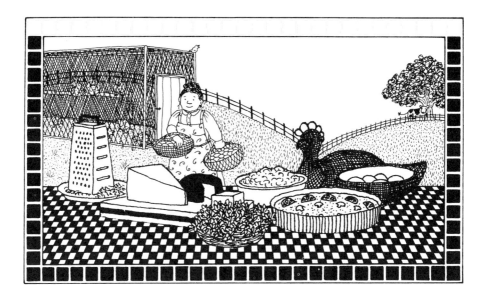

EGGS IN THE MICROWAVE

When eggs are cooked conventionally, they cook from the white in toward the yolk. When eggs are microwaved, the opposite happens. There is more fat in the yolk than in the white, so more microwave energy is attracted to the yolk, and it starts cooking first. Consequently, if the egg is microwaved until the white is completely set, the yolk will be overcooked and will become tough. Therefore, aftercooking time is necessary to finish cooking the white while preventing the yolk from becoming tough.

When you scramble eggs, they cook more evenly because the whites and the yolks are mixed together. Aftercooking time is still necessary to ensure the eggs are cooked sufficiently.

Never microwave an egg still in its shell. Steam builds up under the shell and causes the egg to burst. Hard-cooked eggs can be cooked in small bowls out of the shells and be used in recipes calling for hard-boiled eggs.

POACHED EGGS

SERVING FOR 1

Break 2 eggs into 2 custard cups or use 2 sections of a microwave-safe muffin pan. Cover and microwave at High for 30 seconds. Reduce power to Medium (70%) and microwave for 30 seconds. Allow 2 to 3 minutes aftercooking time.

SERVING FOR 2

Break 4 eggs into 4 custard cups or use 4 sections of a microwave-safe muffin pan. Cover and microwave at High for 1 minute. Reduce power to Medium (70%) and microwave for 40 to 60 seconds. Allow 2 to 3 minutes aftercooking time.

HARD-COOKED EGGS

Line each section of a microwave-safe muffin pan with a paper liner. Break an egg into each section. Cover with microwave-safe plastic wrap. Microwave at Medium (70%) for 2 minutes. Reduce power to Low (30%) and microwave for 6 minutes. Allow 10 minutes aftercooking time. Carefully remove paper liners and place eggs on a paper towel or tea towel until completely cooled. Use in any recipe calling for hard-boiled eggs.

Note: Times may vary depending on the size of the eggs being used as well as the starting temperature of the eggs. All recipes were tested with large eggs straight out of the refrigerator. The cooking pattern in some microwave ovens may make it necessary to pierce the yolks before cooking, to prevent them from popping.

MICROWAVED BACON AND EGGS

Yes, you can serve bacon and eggs cooked in the microwave oven!

....

| 2 | **strips bacon** | 2 |
| 2 | **eggs** | 2 |

....

Preheat a browning skillet for 2 minutes at High. Cut strips of bacon in half crosswise and place in the bottom of the browning skillet around the outside edge. Cover and microwave at High for 2 minutes. Break eggs into the skillet and baste with bacon fat. Cover and microwave at Medium (70%) for 1 to 2 minutes for a hard yolk, or microwave at Medium (70%) for 40 seconds, then reduce power to Medium Low (50%) for 20 to 30 seconds for a soft yolk. Allow 1 to 2 minutes aftercooking time in the browning skillet.

Note: When cooking eggs in the microwave oven, it may sometimes be necessary to prick the yolks with a fork before microwaving in order to prevent popping. Reducing the power level may make pricking unnecessary. Check with the manufacturer's directions.

....

MAKES   1 serving

....

2 PROTEIN CHOICES   14 g protein
2 FATS AND OILS CHOICES   13 g fat
                            155 calories

MICROWAVED EGG SANDWICH

Quick—and easy enough for a child to make for a meal or a snack.

1	egg	1
2	slices bread	2

Toast two slices of bread. Put one slice of toast on a piece of paper towel or tea towel on a microwave-safe plate. Break an egg on top of the toast. Break the yolk, if desired. Top with second slice of toast. Microwave at Medium (70%) for 1 minute. Flip over onto another plate as this plate will be moist, and remove the towelling.

MAKES 1 serving

2 STARCHY CHOICES   30 g carbohydrates
1 PROTEIN CHOICE   9 g protein
                         3 g fat
                         191 calories

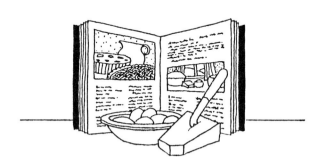

EXTRA-MOIST SCRAMBLED EGGS

These eggs are guaranteed to come out moist and fluffy every time!
Cottage cheese provides a delightful addition.

2	eggs	2
5 mL	water	1 tsp
15 mL	cottage cheese	1 tbsp
5 mL	chopped green onion	1 tsp

Combine eggs and water in a 500 mL (2-cup) measure. Beat with a fork.
Microwave at Medium (70%) for 50 to 70 seconds or until egg is fluffy,
stirring once during cooking. Stir in cottage cheese. Place egg on serving
dish and top with green onion.

MAKES	2 servings
EACH SERVING	1/2 of recipe

1 PROTEIN CHOICE	1 g carbohydrates
1/2 FATS AND OILS CHOICE	7 g protein
	5.5 g fat
	90 calories

EGG SALAD

This Egg Salad is a real hit with my four children.

4	eggs	4
25 mL	chopped green onions	2 tbsp
25 mL	chopped celery	2 tbsp
75 mL	Buttermilk Mayonnaise	1/3 cup
2 mL	dry mustard	1/2 tsp

Break eggs into microwave-safe mug or custard cup. Beat with a fork and cover. Microwave at High for 20 seconds, then at Medium (70%) for 1 to 1-1/2 minutes. Stir. Allow 2 minutes aftercooking time. Combine eggs with onions, celery, mayonnaise and dry mustard, mixing well.

MAKES	4 servings
EACH SERVING	75 mL (1/3 cup)

1 PROTEIN CHOICE	3 g carbohydrates
1 EXTRA CHOICE	7 g protein
1/2 FATS AND OILS CHOICE	5 g fat
	98 calories

EGGS BENEDICT

To serve for that special breakfast.

1	egg yolk	1
175 mL	plain low-fat yogurt	3/4 cup
25 mL	lemon juice	2 tbsp
1 mL	salt	1/4 tsp
0.5 mL	dry mustard	1/8 tsp
6	eggs	6
3	English muffins, split	3
6	slices ham	6
	Parsley as garnish (optional)	

In a small bowl, lightly beat egg yolk. Add 50 mL (1/4 cup) yogurt, lemon juice, salt and mustard. Microwave at High for 30 to 50 seconds, until thick and smooth. Gradually add remaining yogurt, blending well. If more time is needed to thicken, microwave at High for 20 to 30 seconds. Set aside.

Break eggs into individual custard cups or sections of a microwave-safe muffin pan or egg poacher. Cover and microwave at Medium (70%) for 4 to 5 minutes or until eggs are nearly set. Allow 2 to 3 minutes aftercooking time.

Meanwhile, toast split English muffins. Place toasted muffin halves on plates, top with 1 slice of ham, then poached egg. Pour on 25 mL (2 tbsp) of Hollandaise Sauce. Garnish with parsley, if desired.

MAKES	3 or 6 servings	

LARGE SERVING	2 muffin halves	
2 STARCHY CHOICES		32 g carbohydrates
4 PROTEIN CHOICES		30 g protein
1 FATS AND OILS CHOICE		21 g fat
		451 calories

SMALL SERVING	1 muffin half	
1 STARCHY CHOICE		16 g carbohydrates
2 PROTEIN CHOICES		15 g protein
1/2 FATS AND OILS CHOICE		10 g fat
		225 calories

PUFFY OMELETTE

A favorite in my basic microwave cooking class.

4	eggs	4
50 mL	milk	1/4 cup
2 mL	salt	1/2 tsp
1 mL	baking powder	1/4 tsp
0.5 mL	pepper	1/8 tsp
15 mL	butter, margarine OR bacon fat	1 tbsp

Separate eggs, placing whites in a 2 L (2-quart) bowl and yolks in a smaller bowl. Beat egg whites until stiff but not dry. The egg whites should not fall out if the bowl is turned upside down. Blend together yolks, milk, salt, baking powder and pepper. Gently fold yolk mixture into beaten egg whites, using a rubber spatula.

Melt butter in a pie plate at High for 30 to 45 seconds. Pour in eggs. Microwave at Medium Low (50%) for 3 to 5 minutes, until partially set. Lift edges of omelette with a spatula so uncooked portion spreads evenly. Microwave at Medium Low (50%) for 2-1/2 to 4-1/2 minutes, or until centre is almost set. Do not overcook, or the omelette will fall and become rubbery.

Sprinkle desired filling over 1/2 of omelette, then loosen with a spatula and fold in half. Or sprinkle filling over entire omelette and serve in wedges. Omelette may be microwaved at High for 30 to 60 seconds to heat filling. Allow 1 to 2 minutes aftercooking time.

SUGGESTED FILLINGS:

Shredded cheese, crumbled bacon, sliced cooked mushrooms, chopped ham, chopped green pepper, chopped green onion, sautéed onion slices, chopped tomato, diced cooked potato, shredded chipped beef, chopped cooked shrimp

MAKES	2 to 4 servings
EACH SERVING	1/2 omelette for 2 servings
	1/4 omelette for 4 servings

1/2 OMELETTE	
2 PROTEIN CHOICES	14 g protein
	7 g fat
	110 calories

1/4 OMELETTE

1 PROTEIN CHOICE   7 g protein

3 g fat

55 calories

Do not forget to include choices for whatever fillings are used.

QUICHE LORRAINE

Crustless quiche with the taste of the rich version.
A traditional dish at the Empringham clan Christmas dinner.

4	slices bacon	4
375 mL	grated Cheddar cheese	1-1/2 cups
50 mL	chopped onion	1/4 cup
500 mL	skim milk	2 cups
3	eggs	3
2 mL	salt	1/2 tsp
0.5 mL	cayenne	1/8 tsp

Place bacon slices on a microwave-safe rack and cover with a paper towel or parchment paper. Microwave at High for 3 to 4 minutes or until crisp. Crumble into a pie plate with grated cheese and onions.

Combine milk, eggs, salt and cayenne. Whisk until well mixed. Pour over bacon mixture. Microwave at Medium (70%) for 8 to 10 minutes or until centre is partially set. Allow 5 minutes aftercooking time. A knife inserted in the centre should come out clean. If additional cooking is needed, microwave at Medium (70%) for 30-second intervals.

MAKES   6 servings
EACH SERVING   1/6 wedge

2 PROTEIN CHOICES   16 g protein

1 FATS AND OILS CHOICE   11 g fat

155 calories

CHEDDAR CHEESE SAVORY

This hearty brunch dish serves up easily any time. Its preparation is simple and the results are quite tasty.

2	MacIntosh apples, sliced	2
5 mL	lemon juice	1 tsp
4	slices toast	4
250 mL	grated Cheddar cheese	1 cup
	Pepper	

In a small bowl, combine sliced apples and lemon juice. Microwave at High for 2 to 3 minutes or until apples are tender. Spread apples on toast and top with cheese. Microwave at High for 30 to 45 seconds to melt cheese. Sprinkle with pepper and serve.

MAKES 4 servings

EACH SERVING 1 slice of toast plus 1/4 of spread and cheese

1 STARCHY CHOICE	25 g carbohydrates
1 PROTEIN CHOICE	9.4 g protein
1 FRUITS AND VEGETABLES CHOICE	11.5 g fat
1-1/2 FATS AND OILS CHOICES	230 calories

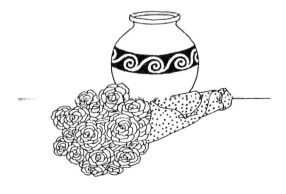

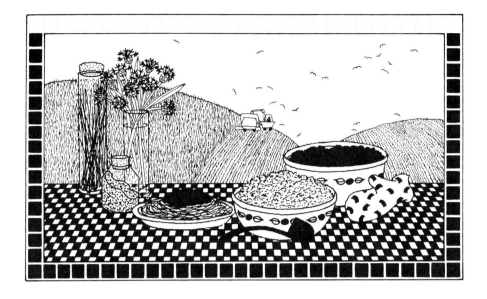

MICROWAVING PASTA

Pasta cooked in your microwave oven takes approximately the same cooking time as conventional methods. It is the absorption of the heated water that softens the pasta. The texture of pasta cooked in the microwave is perfect "al dente." The advantages to microwaving pasta are less heat in the kitchen, easier clean-up and better texture. Since no significant time is saved by cooking pasta in the microwave, it may be better time management to cook the pasta on the stove while you make the sauce in the microwave.

A large casserole should be used to prevent the water from boiling over. Liquids double in volume when boiling in the microwave, so there should be sufficient room in the casserole to allow for this. If allowed to boil over, water will collect around the casserole dish and attract the microwave energy. This will in turn take microwave energy away from the water around the pasta and increase the cooking time. To prevent a build-up of excess moisture, place a terrycloth tea towel around the base of the casserole to absorb this moisture. The microwave energy will be less attracted to the dispersed moisture in the towel than to pools of water.

Place the pasta in the casserole and pour in very hot water until it is 1.25 to 2.5 cm (1/2 to 1 in) above the pasta. Add a few drops of oil and stir. Cover the casserole with a lid—not plastic wrap—and microwave first at High, then at Medium, according to the following chart.

PASTA	HIGH	MEDIUM (70%)
SPAGHETTI	8 to 10 min.	8 to 10 min.
LINGUINE	6 to 8 min.	5 to 6 min.
ROTINI	6 to 8 min.	6 to 8 min.
MANICOTTI (Brush with oil before putting into water)	10 min.	10 min.
LASAGNA	8 to 10 min.	8 to 10 min.
EGG NOODLES	4 to 6 min.	5 to 6 min.
ELBOW MACARONI	7 to 8 min.	7 to 8 min.
SPECIALTY NOODLES	7 to 8 min.	9 to 10 min.

Starting off at High and reducing to Medium allows the temperature of the water to rise rapidly without boiling over and also keeps the temperature high enough to allow the pasta to cook. Stir or rearrange the pasta after the High cooking time and once during the Medium cooking time. After cooking, drain the pasta and rinse with cold water to stop the cooking process. Drain well before serving. The best-textured pasta is cooked to the tender-firm stage called "al dente."

If the pasta cools down, it can be reheated at High for 30 to 60 seconds per 250 mL (1 cup). This timing can also be used after draining to eliminate excess water and make the sauce stick better to the pasta. Place the pasta in a microwave-safe serving dish and microwave.

When the pasta is to be used in a casserole that requires further cooking, it is best to undercook by 2 to 4 minutes when precooking. Leftover pasta can be frozen; when reheated it tastes like a fresh-made dish. (A few drops of water may be needed to freshen it up.) Precooked pasta stored in the freezer will save you lots of time.

When converting conventional recipes to the microwave method, precook the pasta first.

MICROWAVING RICE

Because it is a dry food, rice needs to be rehydrated while cooking. This takes the same amount of time in the microwave as on the stove. Microwaved rice does not burn or stick, and clean-up is easy.

The casserole used for microwaving rice should be large enough to allow room for the water to boil and to prevent boiling over; a guide is a 3 L (3-quart) casserole for 250 to 375 mL (1 to 1-1/2 cups) of rice.

Use the same amount of water as for conventional methods of cooking rice, since rice requires the same amount of water to rehydrate no matter what cooking method is used. Use very hot water. Cold water requires a longer cooking time. To hasten the absorption of the water, cover the casserole, preferably with the lid. Do not use plastic wrap—the contents will become extremely hot and may create a suction under the plastic wrap, making it difficult to remove. To avoid hot steam, always lift the cover from the side furthest from you.

Allow 10 minutes aftercooking time to let the rice finish absorbing the water, then toss with a fork. Remember that aftercooking does not have to be done in the microwave oven. During this time, another dish can be cooked in the microwave.

Frozen rice reheats beautifully, without drying or changing in texture. Defrost rice for 5 minutes per 250 mL (1 cup) before microwaving at High. Sprinkle a little water onto the rice before heating; 250 mL (1 cup) of rice requires 1 to 2 minutes at High to reach serving temperature. Precooked rice stored in the freezer will save you lots of time.

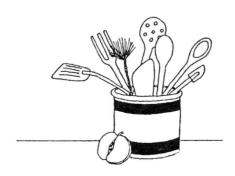

PASTA PRIMAVERA

Pasta is a passion of mine and I need to consume it at least once a day. This recipe lets me eat a generous serving and be comfortable knowing it is low-calorie and healthy!

250 g	thin spaghetti	8 oz
250 mL	broccoli florets	1 cup
250 mL	sliced zucchini	1 cup
250 mL	sliced mushrooms	1 cup
5 mL	basil	1 tsp
2 mL	freshly ground pepper	1/2 tsp
25 mL	grated Parmesan cheese	2 tbsp

Place spaghetti in an oblong baking dish. Cover with water. Microwave at High for 10 to 15 minutes or until water boils. Allow to stand until desired degree of doneness. Drain. In a 2 L (2-quart) casserole, combine broccoli, zucchini and mushrooms with basil and pepper. Microwave at High for 8 to 10 minutes or until vegetables are fork tender. Toss vegetables with spaghetti and top with cheese. Reheat if necessary at High for 3 to 4 minutes.

MAKES	4 servings
EACH SERVING	300 mL (1-1/4 cups)

1 STARCHY CHOICE	21 g carbohydrates
1/2 FRUITS AND VEGETABLES CHOICE	5 g protein
	1 g fat
	120 calories

MEATLESS CHILI AND PASTA

This recipe allows you to cut down on the grocery bill yet still eat a filling meal. My family of six gobbles up this dish in no time—without missing the meat.

250 g	uncooked elbow macaroni	8 oz
1	green pepper, chopped	1
1	onion, chopped	1
500 mL	canned kidney beans	2 cups
125 mL	frozen or canned corn	1/2 cup
250 mL	canned tomatoes	1 cup
2 mL	freshly ground pepper	1/2 tsp
125 mL	grated Cheddar cheese	1/2 cup

Place elbow macaroni in a 2 L (2-quart) casserole. Cover with hot tap water. Microwave at High for 5 to 6 minutes, then at Medium (70%) for 6 minutes. Set aside until Macaroni is al dente. Drain. To macaroni, add green pepper, onion, kidney beans, corn, tomatoes and pepper. Cover with lid or microwave-safe plastic wrap. Microwave at High for 10 minutes, then a Medium (70%) for 10 minutes. Sprinkle with cheese and let stand until cheese is melted.

MAKES	6 servings
EACH SERVING	250 mL (1 cup)

1 STARCHY CHOICE	32 g carbohydrates
1 PROTEIN CHOICE	12 g protein
1 MILK CHOICE	7 g fat
1 FRUITS AND VEGETABLES CHOICE	241 calories
1/2 FATS AND OILS CHOICE	

LASAGNA

A little more work than the higher-calorie version, but well worth the effort.

500 g	lean ground beef	1 lb
2	cloves garlic	2
1	medium onion, chopped	1
1	can (796 mL / 28 oz) stewed tomatoes	1
125 mL	water	1/2 cup
50 mL	tomato paste	1/4 cup
15 mL	parsley	1 tbsp
	Salt to taste	
2 mL	oregano	1/2 tsp
2 mL	thyme	1/2 tsp
2 mL	basil	1/2 tsp
1 mL	ground cloves	1/4 tsp
1 mL	pepper	1/4 tsp
250 mL	2% milk	1 cup
15 mL	flour	1 tbsp
5 mL	cornstarch	1 tsp
2 mL	salt	1/2 tsp
5 mL	vegetable oil	1 tsp
75 mL	grated Parmesan cheese	1/3 cup
9	uncooked lasagna noodles	9
250 g	grated Mozzarella cheese	8 oz
15 mL	grated Parmesan cheese	1 tbsp

Place ground beef in a plastic colander set in a pie plate. Microwave at High for 3 to 5 minutes, stirring occasionally. Spoon meat into a 2 L (2-quart) casserole. Stir in garlic and onion. Microwave at High for 2 to 3 minutes or until onions are limp and beef is no longer pink. Blend in tomatoes, water, tomato paste, and seasoning. Microwave at High 3 to 4 minutes or until boiling. Reduce power to Medium Low (50%) for 5 to 8 minutes.

In a 1 L (1-quart) measure, combine milk, flour, cornstarch and salt. Whisk until completely mixed with no dry bits of cornstarch or flour. Microwave at High for 2 to 3 minutes, stirring every minute, until mixture comes to a boil and thickens. Stir in oil and Parmesan cheese.

In an oblong dish, spread a thin layer of meat sauce. Top with alternating layers of noodles, Parmesan sauce, Mozzarella cheese, and meat sauce, making 3 layers of each and ending with remaining meat sauce. Microwave, covered, at High for 8 minutes. Reduce power to Medium Low (50%) and microwave, covered, for 32 minutes. Top with remaining 15 mL (1 tbsp) Parmesan cheese and allow 15 to 20 minutes aftercooking time, covered, before serving.

MAKES   9 servings

EACH SERVING   one 7.5 × 10 cm (3 × 4 in) piece

3 PROTEIN CHOICES	15 g carbohydrates
1 STARCHY CHOICE	21 g protein
1 FATS AND OILS CHOICE	13 g fat
	261 calories

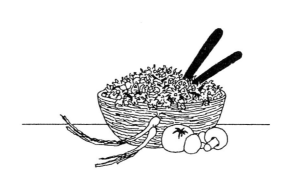

MEATLESS SPAGHETTI SAUCE

Serve with meatballs over noodles or as is with cooked chicken and rice. This sauce can be the base for many Italian recipes.

5 mL	vegetable oil	1 tsp
2	cloves garlic, chopped	2
1	medium onion, chopped	1
1	can (796 mL / 28 oz) stewed tomatoes	1
125 mL	water	1/2 cup
50 mL	tomato paste	1/4 cup
15 mL	dried parsley	1 tbsp
5 mL	salt	1 tsp
2 mL	oregano	1/2 tsp
2 mL	thyme	1/2 tsp
2 mL	basil	1/2 tsp
1 mL	ground cinnamon	1/4 tsp
1 mL	pepper	1/4 tsp

Combine oil, garlic and onion in a 2 L (2-quart) casserole. Microwave at High for 1 to 2 minutes or until onions are limp. Stir in tomatoes, water and tomato paste. Add parsley, salt, oregano, thyme, basil, cinnamon and pepper. Stir well. Microwave at High for 5 to 8 minutes or until boiling. Reduce power to Medium Low (50%) and microwave for 15 minutes, stirring occasionally.

MAKES	6 servings
EACH SERVING	125 mL (1/2 cup)

1 FRUITS AND VEGETABLES CHOICE	9 g carbohydrates
	2 g protein
	1 g fat
	53 calories

CREAMY CHEESE AND MACARONI

This old standby can be made into a seasoned gourmet delight by using sharp cheese and adding a dash of onion powder and a drop of Tabasco sauce.

300 mL	uncooked macaroni	1-1/4 cups
10 mL	margarine	2 tsp
25 mL	flour	2 tbsp
500 mL	skim milk	2 cups
2 mL	salt	1/2 tsp
pinch	pepper	pinch
375 mL	grated Cheddar cheese	1-1/2 cups
25 mL	dry bread crumbs	2 tbsp

In a large casserole, combine macaroni with enough water to cover and "swim." Cover and microwave at High for 6 minutes; reduce power to Medium (70%) and microwave for 6 minutes. Allow 5 minutes aftercooking time, then drain.

Meanwhile, melt margarine in a 1 L (1-quart) measure at High for 30 to 45 seconds. Whisk in flour. Measure milk into a measuring cup and microwave at High for 45 to 60 seconds. Gradually add milk to flour mixture. Stir in salt and pepper. Microwave at Medium (70%) for 3 to 5 minutes, stirring once after 2 minutes. Mixture should come to a boil. Add cheese and mix to melt the cheese. If needed, microwave at High for 30 to 60 seconds to finish melting cheese.

Combine cheese sauce and macaroni in a 1.5 L (1.5-quart) casserole and microwave at Medium (70%) for 5 to 8 minutes. Sprinkle with dry bread crumbs and allow 5 to 10 minutes aftercooking time.

MAKES	4 servings
EACH SERVING	250 mL (1 cup)

2 PROTEIN CHOICES	33 g carbohydrates
2 STARCHY CHOICES	19 g protein
1/2 MILK CHOICE	16 g fat
1-1/2 FATS AND OILS CHOICES	347 calories

BEEF MACARONI DINNER

A meal in itself.

250 mL	uncooked macaroni	1 cup
500 g	lean ground beef	1 lb
250 mL	tomato sauce	1 cup
125 mL	grated Cheddar cheese	1/2 cup
75 mL	frozen corn	1/3 cup
15 mL	dried minced onion	1 tbsp
500 mL	frozen green beans	2 cups
1 mL	salt	1/4 tsp
15 mL	Worcestershire sauce	1 tbsp
2 mL	basil	1/2 tsp

In a large casserole, combine uncooked macaroni with enough hot water to allow the macaroni to "swim." Microwave, covered, at High for 6 to 8 minutes or until water comes to a boil. Reduce power to medium (70%) and microwave for another 6 to 8 minutes. Drain and set aside.

Place ground beef in a plastic colander set in a pie plate. Microwave at High for 6 to 8 minutes. Spoon meat into a 3 L (3-quart) casserole. Add macaroni and remaining ingredients. Mix well. Microwave, covered, at High for 5 minutes. Reduce power to Medium (70%) and microwave, covered, for 15 minutes, stirring 3 or 4 times during cooking. Allow 5 to 10 minutes aftercooking time, covered.

MAKES	6 servings
EACH SERVING	250 mL (1 cup)

1 STARCHY CHOICE	25 g carbohydrates
2 PROTEIN CHOICES	17 g protein
1 FRUITS AND VEGETABLES CHOICE	11 g fat
1 FATS AND OILS CHOICE	267 calories

LONG GRAIN RICE

| 250 mL | long grain rice | 1 cup |
| 500 mL | very hot water | 2 cups |

Combine rice and water in a 3 L (3-quart) casserole. Cover and microwave at High for 12 to 14 minutes, stirring halfway through the cooking time. Allow 10 minutes aftercooking time, covered.

MAKES 8 servings
EACH SERVING 125 mL (1/2 cup)

1 STARCHY CHOICE 15 g carbohydrates

2 g protein

68 calories

INSTANT RICE

| 375 mL | instant rice | 1-1/2 cups |
| 375 mL | very hot water | 1-1/2 cups |

Combine rice and water in a 2 L (2-quart) casserole. Cover and microwave at High for 3 to 4 minutes. Allow 5 minutes aftercooking time, covered.

MAKES 4 servings
EACH SERVING 125 mL (1/2 cup)

1 STARCHY CHOICE 15 g carbohydrates

2 g protein

68 calories

BROWN RICE

Brown rice retains both the bran and germ of the rice kernel. It has a nutty flavor and takes longer to cook than white rice. The "stir frying" in oil softens the bran and germ, preparing it to rehydrate during the cooking time.

15 mL	oil OR margarine	1 tbsp
250 mL	brown rice	1 cup
500 mL	water	2 cups

Place oil or margarine in a 1 L (1-quart) casserole. Microwave at High for 30 to 45 seconds or until hot. Stir rice into oil until coated. Microwave at High for 1-1/2 to 2 minutes or until rice begins to toast. Add water. Cover. Microwave at High for 4 to 5 minutes, then at Low (30%) for 8 to 10 minutes or until most of the water is absorbed. Allow 5 minutes aftercooking time.

MAKES	4 servings
EACH SERVING	125 mL (1/2 cup)

1 STARCHY CHOICE	15 g carbohydrates
1/2 FATS AND OILS CHOICE	2.1 g protein
	3.6 g fat
	90 calories

WILD AND BROWN RICE

Wild rice is not a grain at all, but a grass. It tends to be expensive because it is scarce and difficult to grow commercially. It is still harvested in Canada just as the native Indians have always harvested it—in canoes paddled along the edge of the rice bed.

15 mL	oil OR margarine	1 tbsp
125 mL	brown rice	1/2 cup
125 mL	wild rice	1/2 cup
625 mL	hot tap water	2-1/2 cups
1	clove garlic, minced	1

In a 1 L (1-quart) casserole, microwave oil or margarine at High for 30 to 45 seconds or until hot. Stir in brown and wild rice, and continue to stir until rice is coated. Microwave at High for 1-1/2 to 2 minutes or until rice begins to toast. Add water and garlic. Cover. Microwave at High for 5 to 6 minutes, then at Low (30%) for 10 to 15 minutes or until most of the water is absorbed. Allow 5 minutes aftercooking time. If water remains in the dish, microwave at High for 2 to 3 minutes. Allow to stand again.

MAKES	4 servings
EACH SERVING	125 mL (1/2 cup)

1 STARCHY CHOICE	15 g carbohydrates
1/2 FATS AND OILS CHOICE	2.1 g protein
	3.6 g fat
	90 calories

CHINESE FRIED RICE

"Fried" doesn't always indicate high-fat and stovetop cooking. Microwave "frying" is achieved without slaving over the heat and with little or no fat. Check out the other "fried" recipes in this cookbook—Fried Green Peppers (p. 163), Herbed Chicken Strips (p. 92).

500 mL	hot tap water	2 cups
250 mL	long grain rice	1 cup
45 mL	soya sauce	3 tbsp
50 mL	frozen peas	1/4 cup
1	egg	1

In a 1 L (1-quart) dish, combine water and rice. Microwave at High for 4 to 5 minutes, then simmer at Low (30%) for 6 to 8 minutes or until most of the water is absorbed. Allow to stand. While rice is still hot, stir in soya sauce and frozen peas until well combined. Add egg and stir to coat rice. Microwave at High for 30 to 45 seconds to thoroughly cook the egg.

MAKES	4 servings
EACH SERVING	125 mL (1/2 cup)

2 STARCHY CHOICES	27 g carbohydrates
1/2 FATS AND OILS CHOICE	5 g protein
	2 g fat
	147 calories

CURRIED RICE

This rice makes a great side dish for chicken or pork. It's a beautiful yellow and tastes as good as it looks. Select the curry powder according to your taste—mild, medium or hot.

250 mL	hot tap water	1 cup
250 mL	chicken broth	1 cup
250 mL	long grain rice	1 cup
50 mL	raisins	1/4 cup
5 mL	curry powder	1 tsp
2 mL	garlic powder	1/2 tsp
2 mL	dried parsley	1/2 tsp

In a 1 L (1-quart) casserole, combine all ingredients. Stir. Cover and cook at High for 4 to 5 minutes, then at Low (30%) for 6 to 8 minutes or until most of the water is absorbed. Allow 5 minutes aftercooking time.

MAKES	4 servings
EACH SERVING	125 mL (1/2 cup)

2 STARCHY CHOICES

36 g carbohydrates

2.1 g protein

140 calories

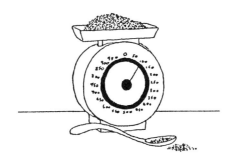

RICE PILAF

Stir in heated leftover meat for a complete meal. Leftovers heated in the microwave taste as good as the original meal.

250 mL	long grain rice	1 cup
15 mL	vegetable oil	1 tbsp
50 mL	finely chopped celery	1/4 cup
50 mL	chopped green onion	1/4 cup
500 mL	water	2 cups
10 mL	chicken or beef bouillon concentrate	2 tsp
75 mL	sliced mushrooms	1/3 cup

In a 1.5 L (1.5-quart) casserole, combine rice and vegetable oil. Microwave at High for 2 to 3 minutes, stirring once. Stir in celery and green onions. Microwave at High for 1 minute. Add water and bouillon. Mix well and cover. Microwave at High for 5 minutes, then at Medium Low (50%) for 16 to 18 minutes. Stir in mushrooms. Allow 10 minutes aftercooking time, covered. Fluff with a fork.

MAKES   8 servings

EACH SERVING   125 mL (1/2 cup)

1 STARCHY CHOICE   21 g carbohydrates

1/2 FRUITS AND VEGETABLES CHOICE   3 g protein

                                                  2 g fat

                                                  120 calories

RISOTTO PARMESAN

Rice, pasta and potatoes can get so boring! Try this recipe and your own variations. Add mint or oregano, use tomato juice (an Extra choice) instead of bouillon, or add chopped mushrooms or celery.

....

50 mL	chopped onion	1/4 cup
375 mL	white rice	1-1/2 cups
750 mL	chicken bouillon	3 cups
50 mL	grated Parmesan cheese	1/4 cup

....

Place onions in a 2 L (2-quart) casserole. Microwave at High for 30 to 45 seconds or until onion begins to soften. Stir in rice and bouillon. Cover. Microwave at High for 6 to 7 minutes or until boiling. Reduce power to Medium Low (50%) and microwave for 8 to 10 minutes or until most of the water is absorbed. Stir in cheese. Cover. Allow 5 minutes aftercooking time.

....

MAKES	4 full-course or 8 side-dish servings
EACH SERVING	Side dish—100 mL (1/3 cup plus 2 tbsp)
	Full course—200 mL (1/2 cup plus 1/3 cup)

....

SIDE DISH

1 STARCHY CHOICE	19 g carbohydrates
1 EXTRA CHOICE	2.6 g protein
	97 calories

....

FULL COURSE

2 STARCHY CHOICES	39 g carbohydrates
1 FRUITS AND VEGETABLES CHOICE	5.3 g protein
	195 calories

MINTY RICE AND VEGETABLES

This tasty dish makes a special dish to serve on a buffet or to company. The color is vibrant and its flavor has a delightful freshness.

15 mL	vegetable oil	1 tbsp
250 mL	brown rice	1 cup
500 mL	warm water	2 cups
2	onions, sliced	2
1	clove garlic, minced	1
1	celery stalk, sliced	1
250 mL	broccoli florets	1 cup
2	carrots, sliced	2
1	red pepper, chopped	1
5 mL	mint	1 tsp
50 mL	chicken bouillon	1/4 cup
125 mL	plain yogurt	1/2 cup

In 2 L (2-quart) casserole, microwave oil at High for 30 seconds. Add rice and microwave at High for 1-1/2 minutes. Stir. Pour in water. Cover tightly. Microwave at High for 6 to 7 minutes or until boiling. Reduce power to Medium Low (50%) for 12 to 15 minutes. Add onions, garlic, celery, broccoli, carrots, red pepper, mint and bouillon to the rice, stirring well. Cover and microwave at High for 7 minutes or until vegetables are fork tender. Stir in yogurt. Allow 5 minutes aftercooking time, covered.

MAKES	4 servings
EACH SERVING	425 mL (1-3/4 cups)

1 STARCHY CHOICE	22 g carbohydrates
1 FRUITS AND VEGETABLES CHOICE	4 g protein
1 FATS AND OILS CHOICE	4 g fat
	141 calories

BARLEY SIDE-DISH

Barley seems to appear in soups and little else. Try this side dish instead of potatoes, rice or noodles for a change. It is nice served with beef or chicken. Whole barley is often called pot barley and is darker, sweeter and nuttier than pearl barley, which is white.

250 mL	whole barley	1 cup
750 mL	water	3 cups
5 mL	thyme	1 tsp
2 mL	sage	1/2 tsp
5 mL	chicken bouillon powder	1 tsp

In a 1 L (1-quart) casserole, combine all ingredients. Cover. Microwave at High for 6 to 8 minutes or until boiling. Continue to cook at Medium Low (50%) for 10 to 15 minutes or until barley is tender. Allow to stand covered to absorb remaining water.

MAKES	8 servings
EACH SERVING	90 mL (1/3 cup plus 1 tbsp)

1 STARCHY CHOICE	19 g carbohydrates
1 EXTRA CHOICE	2 g protein
	87 calories

CRACKED WHEAT

The cracked wheat used in this recipe is properly called bulgur—kernels of whole wheat crushed and parboiled. Bulgur cooks faster than cracked wheat.

....

250 mL	bulgur	1 cup
500 mL	hot tap water	2 cups
5 mL	beef bouillon powder	1 tsp

....

Combine all ingredients in a 1 L (1-quart) casserole. Cover. Microwave at High for 4 to 5 minutes or until boiling. Stir and allow 5 minutes aftercooking time, covered.

....

| **MAKES** | 4 servings |
| **EACH SERVING** | 125 mL (1/2 cup) |

....

2 STARCHY CHOICES	32 g carbohydrates
	5 g protein
	150 calories

HOT CRACKED WHEAT CEREAL

Grains are excellent sources of the B vitamins and phosphorus, magnesium, copper, chromium, manganese and selenium. They have the added benefit of being slowly digested, keeping one feeling full longer and stabilizing blood sugar for a longer period.

250 mL	cracked wheat	1 cup
500 mL	hot tap water	2 cups
15 mL	chopped dates	1 tbsp

Combine all ingredients in a 1 L (1-quart) measure. Microwave at High for 4 to 5 minutes or until boiling. Cover and allow to stand 5 minutes. Serve with topping of milk or plain yogurt.

MAKES   4 servings

EACH SERVING   125 mL (1/2 cup)

2 STARCHY CHOICES   39 g carbohydrates

1 FRUITS AND VEGETABLES CHOICE   5 g protein

130 calories

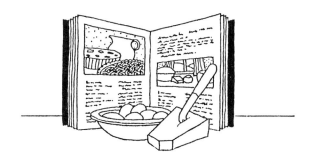

OATMEAL

Oatmeal or porridge has been the traditional hot breakfast for generations. Rolled oats are grains that have been steamed and flattened, and they come in three thicknesses—regular old-fashioned (thickest), quick-cooking oats, and instant oats. This recipe uses quick-cooking oats, so add 30 seconds cooking time if you choose regular old-fashioned oats.

| 250 mL | water | 1 cup |
| 75 mL | rolled oats | 1/3 cup |

In a 500 mL (2-cup) measure, combine water and oats. Microwave at High for 2 to 3 minutes. Stir. Continue to cook at Medium (70%) for 1 to 1-1/2 minutes or until oats are tender. Serve with topping of milk or yogurt.

| MAKES | 2 servings |
| EACH SERVING | 125 mL (1/2 cup) |

1 STARCHY CHOICE

15 g carbohydrates

2 g protein

68 calories

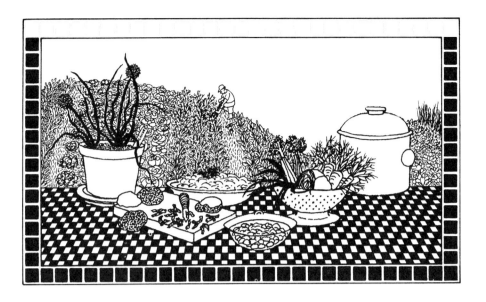

What better way to serve vegetables for the diabetic than microwaved? Picture-perfect vegetables can be obtained without the added calories of sauces. They are beautiful on their own. You may even find you prefer a vegetable microwaved that you did not like when cooked conventionally. The quality and taste are outstanding, since microwaving retains the natural colors, flavors and nutrients. Vegetables can be microwaved to tender-crisp or soft, depending on personal preference.

MICROWAVING VEGETABLES

Most fresh vegetables do not require added water for cooking; usually the water clinging to them after washing is sufficient. Frozen vegetables usually need no added water because the ice crystals provide sufficient liquid. Only vegetables that are dense or tend to be dry should have water added for cooking. Vegetables with a skin, such as potatoes and squash, do not require a container but will need to be pierced to allow steam to escape.

Cut-up vegetables should be of uniform size and shape to allow for even cooking. Do not salt vegetables before cooking, or brown spots will develop and the microwave cooking pattern will be altered. Cover vegetables to be cooked in the microwave either with the casserole lid or waxed paper.

Most fresh vegetables require 6 minutes per 500 g (1 lb) at High.

Exceptions are those with a high water content such as tomatoes and mushrooms. Do not overcook vegetables; they quickly become tough and dried-out. Allow 5 minutes aftercooking time.

Canned vegetables should have the liquid drained, but reserve 15 to 25 mL (1 to 2 tbsp). Pour drained vegetables and reserved liquid into a casserole. Cover. Microwave at High, stirring once or twice.

Frozen vegetables in bulk should be placed in a casserole and covered.

VEGETABLE MICROWAVE COOKING CHART

VEGETABLE	QUANTITY FRESH	SPECIAL INSTRUCTIONS FOR FRESH
ARTICHOKE	1 med.	brush with lemon juice to prevent discoloration, wrap in waxed paper or microwave-safe plastic wrap, place in casserole
ASPARAGUS	500 g	break off bottoms, stand up in a measuring cup, cover with a microwave-safe plastic bag or plastic wrap and secure with an elastic
BEANS	500 g (1 lb) 750 mL (3 cups)	add 50 mL (1/4 cup) water
BEETS	4 med. 500 g (1 lb)	place in 4 L (4-quart) casserole, cover with water, microwave at High for 15 to 17 min.
BROCCOLI	500 g (1 lb)	arrange with the stalks to the outside
BRUSSELS SPROUTS	300 mL (10 oz)	add 25 mL (2 tbsp) water
CABBAGE	500 g (1 lb)	add 25 mL (2 tbsp) water
CARROTS	6 med. 500 g (1 lb)	cut in even-sized pieces, add 50 mL (1/4 cup) water, microwave 7 to 8 min. per 500 g (1 lb)
CAULIFLOWER	500 g (1 lb)	if left whole, wrap in waxed paper

Microwave at High, stirring once or twice to break apart the pieces and to distribute the heat evenly. Allow 5 minutes aftercooking time.

Frozen vegetables in pouches should be flexed to break apart the vegetables. Cut an "X" in the pouch. Place the pouch in a casserole with the cut side down. Microwave at High. Lift the pouch at the corners and allow the vegetables to fall from the pouch into the casserole. Stir, cover, and allow 5 minutes aftercooking time.

QUANTITY FROZEN	SPECIAL INSTRUCTIONS FOR FROZEN	SEASONINGS FOR FRESH OR FROZEN
300 mL (10 oz)	5 to 6 min. High	garlic salt, lemon slices
300 mL (10 oz)	5 to 7 min. High	marjoram, basil, chervil, tarragon, thyme
300 mL (10 oz)	4 to 7 min. High	thyme, savory, tarragon, lemon pepper, dill, oregano, celery seed, rosemary, sage
		celery seed, dill, mint, tarragon, thyme
300 mL (10 oz)	5 to 7 min. High	
300 mL 10 (oz)	5 to 7 min. High	seasoned salt, basil, dill
		basil, dill, savory, sage
500 mL (2 cups)	5 to 7 min. High	nutmeg, marjoram, parsley, mint, basil, thyme, chervil
300 mL (10 oz)	5 to 7 min. High	nutmeg, oregano, rosemary

VEGETABLE	QUANTITY FRESH	SPECIAL INSTRUCTIONS FOR FRESH
CORN	500 mL (2 cups)	
CORN ON THE COB	1 med.	do not husk, remove silk, microwave 2 to 3 min. per cob
EGGPLANT	1 small	dice, add 25 mL (2 tbsp) water, or pierce and cook whole
MUSHROOMS		4 min. per 500 g (1 lb)
ONIONS	8 small 2 large 500 g (1 lb)	whole, sliced or quartered
PARSNIPS	4 med.	add 25 mL (2 tbsp) water, 7 to 8 min. per 500 g (1 lb)
PEAS	500 mL (1 lb)	add 25 mL (2 tbsp) water
PEA PODS	125 g (1/4 lb)	cut off end of pod but leave string attached; pull string down pod, repeat on other end; add 25 mL (2 tbsp) water
SQUASH acorn, butternut	500 g (1 lb)	pierce and put on rack
SQUASH hubbard	500 g (1 lb)	may be cut into cubes, add 25 mL (2 tbsp) water, precook 2 min.
TOMATOES	4 med.	select ripe and firm, and avoid overcooking

QUANTITY FROZEN	SPECIAL INSTRUCTIONS FOR FROZEN	SEASONINGS FOR FRESH OR FROZEN
300 mL (10 oz)	4 to 6 min. High	
1 med.	1 to 2 min. per cob tightly covered with microwave-safe plastic wrap High	
		nutmeg, savory, chervil, marjoram
		thyme, oregano, marjoram, tarragon, rosemary, sage
		caraway seed, thyme, cloves, nutmeg, marjoram, sage
		parsley, nutmeg, cinnamon
300 mL (10 oz)	4 to 6 min. High	savory, marjoram, tarragon, mint, thyme, sage
180 mL	2 to 4 min. High	savory, tarragon, marjoram, mint, thyme, sage
mashed 360 mL (1-1/2 cups)	5 to 8 min., break apart after 2 min. High	savory, nutmeg, basil, dill, marjoram, mint
		savory, nutmeg, basil, dill, marjoram, mint
		celery seed, basil, savory, dill, marjoram, oregano, rosemary, sage

VEGETABLE	QUANTITY FRESH	SPECIAL INSTRUCTIONS FOR FRESH
TURNIPS	2 med. 500 g (1 lb.)	cut in 1/8 pieces, add water, may be done whole with paper towel underneath
YAMS	2 med. 500 g (1 lb)	even-sized pieces on rack

Note: All vegetables should be microwaved covered, whether with a casserole lid or natural cover (skin of vegetable) and microwaved for 6 to 8 minutes per 500 g (1 lb), at High, unless otherwise stated in the chart. Allow 5 minutes aftercooking time. Cooking by weight is an accurate method of determining cooking time. There may be some variations depending on the texture, freshness and shape of the vegetable. The times given in the chart are for tender-crisp vegetables. If a softer vegetable is desired, add another 15 mL (1 tbsp) water and microwave 1 to 2 minutes longer.

BLANCHING FRESH VEGETABLES IN THE MICROWAVE

Using your microwave oven to blanch vegetables before freezing them is an ideal method. A vegetable garden in your backyard will provide young, tender vegetables when they are at their peak of flavor. You can then blanch the vegetables in small batches rather than waiting to blanch a whole crop at one time. Your kitchen will stay cool, and small batches done in the microwave oven will be easier to handle than the steaming pot used for conventional blanching.

Vegetables are blanched to inactivate the enzymes in order to prevent off-flavors and preserve the vitamin content while frozen. Follow the directions in the chart below for the vegetables indicated. For any vegetables not included on the chart, follow directions in your microwave manual for microwaving the fresh vegetable. Be sure not to add salt; this will affect cooking time and evenness. Blanch for one-quarter the regular time. Green vegetables should be blanched only until there is a color change. All other vegetables should be blanched until pliable but not tender. When blanching vegetables in the microwave oven, do not increase the quantities. If you are doing several batches, clean one batch while another batch is microwaving.

QUANTITY FROZEN	SPECIAL INSTRUCTIONS FOR FROZEN	SEASONINGS FOR FRESH OR FROZEN
		caraway seed, oregano, rosemary, savory
		cinnamon, cloves, nutmeg

Method:

1. Clean vegetables in cool water and prepare by slicing or dicing in uniform sizes as desired.

2. Accurately measure amount to be blanched according to Blanching Chart. Pour into a 2 L (2-quart) casserole. Add water if needed, but do not add salt. Cover.

3. Microwave at High for time indicated on the chart, stirring once. Vegetables should be an even color throughout. Drain.

4. Immediately submerse vegetables in ice-cold water to stop the cooking process. Allow to drain after completely cooled. Spread on paper towel or tea towel to absorb excess water.

5. Place in freezer bags, squeezing to remove air. Label and freeze immediately.

6. In order to loose-pack vegetables in large bags, spread individual pieces on a cookie sheet and freeze. When vegetables are frozen, place loose frozen pieces in a freezer bag. Label and return to the freezer.

BLANCHING CHART

VEGETABLE	AMOUNT	WATER	TIME AT HIGH
ASPARAGUS 1 cm (2 in)	500 g (1 lb)	50 mL (1/4 cup)	2 to 3 min.
BEANS green or wax 5 cm (2 in)	500 g (1 lb)	50 mL (1/4 cup)	4 to 6 min.
BROCCOLI 2.5 cm (1 in)	1 bunch	50 mL (1/4 cup)	4 to 5 min.
BRUSSELS SPROUTS	280 g (10 oz)	50 mL (1/4 cup)	3 to 4 min.
CARROTS (sliced)	500 g (1 lb)	125 mL (1/2 cup)	4 to 6 min.
CAULIFLOWER FLORETS	1 head	50 mL (1/4 cup)	3 to 4 min.
CORN (off cob)	4 med.	50 mL (1/4 cup)	3 to 4 min.
ONIONS (quartered)	4 med.	125 mL (1/2 cup)	3 to 4 min.
PEAS	1 kg (2 lb)	50 mL (1/4 cup)	3 to 4 min.
SPINACH	500 g (1 lb)		2 to 3 min.
ZUCCHINI (sliced)	500 g (1 lb)	50 mL (1/4 cup)	3 to 4 min.

BAKED ACORN SQUASH

Many people still insist on cutting up squash and turnips before cooking them in the microwave oven. Try this easy method and never cut another squash or turnip again!

....

1	acorn squash	1
50 mL	crushed pineapple	1/4 cup
dash	cinnamon	dash

....

Pierce squash with fork several times. Microwave at High for 5 to 7 minutes or until fork tender. Cut in half and remove seeds. Scoop out pulp, being careful not to damage shell. Combine pulp with pineapple and cinnamon. Place mixture in shell. If necessary, reheat at High for 1 minute.

....

MAKES   4 servings
EACH SERVING   75 mL (1/3 cup)

....

1 FRUITS AND VEGETABLES CHOICE   10 g carbohydrates

1 g protein

44 calories

GREEN BEANS AMANDINE

Green beans are a nice vegetable to serve for company. Adding nuts makes this version extra special.

50 mL	sliced almonds	1/4 cup
500 mL	sliced green beans	2 cups
5 mL	water	1 tsp

Place almonds in a custard cup. Microwave at High for 2 to 3 minutes or until beginning to brown, stirring several times during toasting. Set aside. In a 500 mL (2-cup) dish, combine green beans and water. Cover. Microwave at High for 4 to 5 minutes. Stir in almonds.

MAKES	4 servings
EACH SERVING	125 mL (1/2 cup)

1/2 FRUITS AND VEGETABLES CHOICE	3.8 g carbohydrates
	1.8 g protein
	2 g fat
	38 calories

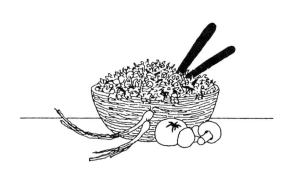

BAKED BEANS

The trend in food is back to basics, including legumes and beans. This recipe sets you in good stead. Oven-baked beans take up to 12 hours to cook, but the microwave oven cuts that time to under 2 hours. Try them soon!

500 mL	dried soy OR navy beans	2 cups
1.5 L	water	6 cups
750 mL	water	3 cups
750 mL	vegetable juice	3 cups
5 mL	dried mustard	1 tsp
125 mL	tomato paste	1/2 cup

Combine dried beans and 1.5 L (6 cups) water and allow to soak overnight. Drain. In a 2.5 L (2.5-quart) casserole, combine beans, 750 mL (3 cups) water and remaining ingredients. Cover. Microwave at High for 20 minutes, then simmer at Medium Low (50%) for 90 minutes. Allow 15 minutes aftercooking time.

MAKES	10 servings
EACH SERVING	125 mL (1/2 cup)

1 STARCHY CHOICE	23 g carbohydrates
1 FRUITS AND VEGETABLES CHOICE	7.6 g protein
1/2 PROTEIN CHOICE	.7 g fat
	124 calories

LEMON BROCCOLI

A nice change from broccoli with cheese sauce.

1	bunch broccoli, about 750 g (1-1/2 lb)	1
25 mL	butter	2 tbsp
25 mL	lemon juice	2 tbsp

Wash broccoli and cut off tough stalks. Cut into even-sized pieces for uniform cooking. Put in 2 L (2-quart) casserole. Cover and microwave at High for 5 to 8 minutes or until done to desired tenderness. Do not overcook; broccoli should be tender-crisp but not limp. During after-cooking, melt butter in small bowl or measuring cup at High for 30 to 45 seconds. Stir in lemon juice. Pour over broccoli and serve.

MAKES	8 servings
EACH SERVING	175 mL (3/4 cup)

1/2 FATS AND OILS CHOICE	5 g fat
1 EXTRA CHOICE	45 calories

CHEF DON'S BROCCOLI AND CAULIFLOWER BEEHIVE

A favorite at all my cooking classes. Many of my students report how impressed their families and friends are when this is served.

1	large head cauliflower	1
2	bunches broccoli	2

Break vegetables into florets and wash them. Line bottom of a batter bowl or flower-pot-shaped mould with cauliflower. Next, make a layer of broccoli, with the stems toward the inside of the dish. Repeat, alternating layers until all the vegetables are used. Cover tightly with microwave-safe plastic wrap. Secure with a rubber band, if necessary.

Microwave at High for 6 minutes for 1 L (1-quart) mould or 12 minutes for 2 L (2-quart) mould. Test for doneness by sticking a skewer into the centre of the mould. Release the steam and compress the vegetables with a saucer. Let cool for about 5 minutes, then drain off the water in the bottom. Place a serving plate over the mould and invert the mould. Remove the mould dish.

Top with Mock Hollandaise Sauce (p. 57), if desired.

....

MAKES   6 to 8 servings

EACH SERVING   125 mL (1/2 cup)

....

1 EXTRA CHOICE

CABBAGE VINAIGRETTE

This idea for preparing cabbage comes from my grandmother of Polish background. I updated the recipe for use in a microwave oven—and not on a wood stove as she used in the past!

....

1/2	head green cabbage	1/2
1	onion, sliced	1
15 mL	wine vinegar	1 tbsp
5 mL	water	1 tsp
2 mL	caraway seeds (optional)	1/2 tsp

....

Slice or shred cabbage. Combine all ingredients in 1 L (1-quart) dish. Cover. Microwave at High for 5 to 6 minutes or until cabbage begins to become limp.

....

MAKES   6 servings

EACH SERVING   125 mL (1/2 cup)

....

1/2 FRUITS AND VEGETABLES CHOICE   4 g carbohydrates

                                                      1 g protein

                                                      18 calories

CARROTS AND APPLES

How do you persuade children to eat vegetables? Serve this recipe often! The color is great (don't peel the apple), and they can help with preparation.

1	apple, diced	1
5	carrots, sliced	5
5 mL	margarine	1 tsp

Combine apple, carrots and margarine in a 1 L (1-quart) casserole. Cover. Microwave at High for 7 to 8 minutes or until carrots are fork tender.

MAKES 4 servings
EACH SERVING 125 mL (1/2 cup)

1-1/2 FRUITS AND VEGETABLES CHOICES

15 g carbohydrates
1 g protein
1.4 g fat
70 calories

DILL CARROTS

Company-style vegetables that are easy and quick enough for every day.

500 g	baby carrots	1 lb
25 mL	butter OR margarine	2 tbsp
1 mL	dillweed	1/4 tsp
1 mL	salt	1/4 tsp
dash	pepper	dash
15 mL	water	1 tbsp

Wash and peel carrots. Cut into strips resembling french fries or slice into evenly-sized coin shapes. Place carrots in a casserole. Dot with butter or margarine and sprinkle with seasonings and water. Cover and microwave at High for 8 to 10 minutes or until carrots are tender-crisp, stirring twice. Allow 5 minutes aftercooking time.

MAKES   5 servings
EACH SERVING   125 mL (1/2 cup)

1 FRUITS AND VEGETABLES CHOICE   15 g carbohydrates
1/2 FATS AND OILS CHOICE   2 g protein
                                       3 g fat
                                       91 calories

CAULIFLOWER AND CARROTS

A colorful display to tantalize the appetite.

375 mL	cauliflower florets	1-1/2 cups
50 mL	water	1/4 cup
250 mL	carrots, cut in 0.5 cm (1/4-in) slices	1 cup

Place cauliflower florets in a pie plate or 1.5 L (1.5-quart) casserole. Add water. Cover and microwave at High for 2 to 3 minutes. Stir in carrots. Cover and microwave at High for 2 to 4-1/2 minutes. Allow 3 to 5 minutes for aftercooking time.

MAKES   4 servings
EACH SERVING   125 mL (1/2 cup)

1/2 FRUITS AND VEGETABLES CHOICE   8.5 g carbohydrates
1 EXTRA CHOICE   36 calories

CAULIFLOWER PLUS

A great way to use a zucchini!

250 mL	2% milk	1 cup
15 mL	all-purpose flour	1 tbsp
5 mL	cornstarch	1 tsp
	Salt to taste	
5 mL	vegetable oil	1 tsp
1	cauliflower	1
1	medium zucchini, sliced	1
3	green onions, chopped	3
1	tomato	1
	grated Parmesan cheese	

In a 1 L (1-quart) measure, combine milk, flour, cornstarch and salt. Whisk until completely mixed with no dry bits of cornstarch or flour. Microwave at High for 2 to 3 minutes, stirring every minute until mixture comes to a boil and thickens. Stir in oil.

Separate cauliflower into florets and place in a casserole. Microwave at High for 5 minutes. Add zucchini and microwave at High for 3 to 4 minutes or until vegetables are tender-crisp. Pour sauce over vegetables and stir to combine. Slice tomato into 8 wedges and arrange on top. Sprinkle lightly with Parmesan cheese. Microwave at High for 3 to 5 minutes or until heated through.

MAKES	4 servings
EACH SERVING	125 mL (1/2 cup) of cauliflower plus 75 mL (1/3 cup) sauce

1 MILK (2%) CHOICE	15 g carbohydrates
1 FRUITS AND VEGETABLES CHOICE	5 g protein
	2 g fat
	91 calories

CHEESY CAULIFLOWER

My children will not eat cauliflower any other way!

1	head cauliflower, about 500 g (1 lb)	1
15 mL	lemon juice	1 tbsp
15 mL	margarine	1 tbsp
15 mL	flour	1 tbsp
125 mL	skim milk	1/2 cup
125 mL	grated Cheddar cheese	1/2 cup
15 mL	parsley	1 tbsp
dash	cayenne	dash

Wash cauliflower, remove leaves and core, and divide into florets. Put cauliflower into 2 L (2-quart) casserole. Sprinkle with lemon juice. Cover and microwave at High for 5 to 8 minutes or until cauliflower is tender-crisp.

In a small bowl or measuring cup, melt margarine at High for 20 to 30 seconds. Blend in flour. In another measure, microwave milk at High for 45 seconds. Gradually combine milk with flour mixture. Add cheese and mix well. If needed, microwave at High for 30 to 45 seconds longer to finish melting the cheese. Pour over cauliflower and sprinkle with cayenne. Allow 3 to 5 minutes for aftercooking time.

MAKES	6 servings
EACH SERVING	150 mL (2/3 cup)

1 EXTRA CHOICE	5 g fat
1 FATS AND OILS CHOICE	45 calories

EGGPLANT PROVENCAL

Purchase eggplant when its skin is smooth and unscarred. Store in the refrigerator and cut off the stem before using.

250 mL	tomatoes, puréed	1 cup
5 mL	oregano	1/2 tsp
2 mL	garlic powder	1/4 tsp
2 mL	freshly ground pepper	1/4 tsp
500 g	eggplant	1 lb
4	lettuce leaves	4
15 mL	chopped parsley	1 tbsp
5 mL	drained capers	1 tsp

Combine tomato purée, oregano, garlic powder and ground pepper. Set aside. Slice eggplant thinly. Arrange eggplant in a 2 L (2-quart) casserole. Cover. Microwave at High for 4 to 5 minutes or until eggplant is transparent.

Place 1 lettuce leaf on each serving dish. Top with 1/4 of eggplant and 50 mL (1/4 cup) tomato sauce. Garnish with parsley and capers.

MAKES	4 servings
EACH SERVING	175 mL (3/4 cup)

1/2 FRUITS AND VEGETABLES CHOICE

6 g carbohydrates

1 g protein

33 calories

FRIED GREEN PEPPERS

Fried green peppers have always been a favorite of mine, and I needed to make them microwaveable. Serve these on a roll for lunch or dinner or by themselves as a snack.

2	green peppers, sliced	2
1	onion, sliced	1
125 mL	sliced mushrooms	1/2 cup
125 mL	tomato sauce	1/2 cup
	Parsley to garnish	

In a 500 mL (2-cup) dish, combine green peppers, onion and mushrooms. Cover. Microwave at High for 4 to 5 minutes. Stir in tomato sauce and continue to Microwave at High for 1 minute. Top with parsley.

MAKES	4 servings
EACH SERVING	125 mL (1/2 cup)

1 EXTRA CHOICE	5 g carbohydrates
	1 g protein
	20 calories

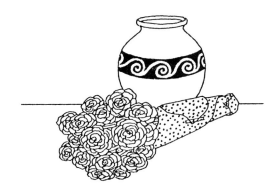

GRAIN-STUFFED PEPPERS

I love dishes that can be prepared ahead of time and cooked when needed. This dish is just that, making it perfect for a party, buffet or a dish to give to a friend.

1	onion, sliced	1
1	clove garlic, minced	1
2	tomatoes, diced	2
2 mL	thyme	1/2 tsp
125 mL	cracked wheat	1/2 cup
	OR bulgur	
250 mL	water	1 cup
50 mL	chopped fresh parsley	3 tbsp
4	green peppers	4

In a 1 L (1-quart) measure, combine onion, garlic and tomatoes and microwave at High for 2 to 3 minutes. Add thyme, cracked wheat and water. Cover and microwave at High for 3 minutes. Let stand until cracked wheat absorbs all the water. Blend in chopped parsley.

Remove stem and seeds from the green peppers. Fill each with 50 mL (1/4 cup) filling. Arrange peppers on a microwave-safe dinner plate and cover with pie plate or microwave-safe plastic wrap. Microwave at High for 4 to 5 minutes or until peppers are tender.

MAKES	4 servings
EACH SERVING	1 stuffed pepper

2 FRUITS AND VEGETABLES CHOICES	38 g carbohydrates
1 STARCHY CHOICE	6 g protein
	1 g fat
	103 calories

BAKED POTATOES

Madame Benoît called these Extra Special Potatoes, and you will find out why! The coating of oil and salt helps the potatoes crisp up in the microwave oven, and the garlic adds a subtle flavor.

4	small potatoes	4
1	clove garlic, minced	1
5 mL	vegetable oil	1 tsp
2 mL	pickling salt	1/2 tsp

Wash and prick potatoes. Combine remaining ingredients in a small bowl. Rub each potato in the mixture to coat lightly. Bake at High for 8 to 10 minutes. Allow 5 minutes aftercooking time.

Note: Potatoes vary greatly in amount of moisture, size and shape. A good rule of thumb is to bake 1 minute per 2.5 cm (1 in) of the potatoes' length.

MAKES	4 servings
EACH SERVING	1 potato

1 STARCHY CHOICE	18 g carbohydrates
1/2 FATS AND OILS CHOICE	2 g protein
	1.3 g fat
	112 calories

POTATO PUFF

Serve this dish in an elegant soufflé dish to impress company! It is a good accompaniment to roast chicken, beef or pork.

6	baking potatoes	6
50 mL	cottage cheese	1/4 cup
25 mL	chopped onion	2 tbsp
125 mL	skim milk	1/2 cup
2	egg whites, beaten until foamy	2
2 mL	tarragon	1/4 tsp
	Paprika	

Place potatoes in a circle on tray of microwave oven. Microwave at High for 12 to 15 minutes. Let stand 5 minutes. Peel potatoes and mash. Whisk cottage cheese until smooth. Combine cheese with onion and milk. Gently fold in egg whites and tarragon. Pour into 1 L (1-quart) microwave-safe soufflé dish. Sprinkle with paprika. Microwave at High for 3 to 4 minutes or until heated through.

MAKES	8 servings
EACH SERVING	125 mL (1/2 cup)

1 STARCHY CHOICE	26 g carbohydrates
1 FRUITS AND VEGETABLES CHOICE	5.4 g protein
	.5 g fat
	127 calories

POTATO AND CABBAGE CASSEROLE

This hearty Irish dish came to me from a friend's mother. She grew up in Ireland, where potatoes are served at each meal of the day. Serve this dish with Turkey Sausage Patties (p. 105) or Saucy Pork Chops (p. 84).

4	potatoes	4
500 mL	shredded cabbage	2 cups
1	onion, chopped	1
50 mL	skim milk	1/4 cup
5 mL	margarine	1 tsp
125 mL	grated Cheddar cheese	1/2 cup
	Pepper to taste	

Wash potatoes. Microwave at High for 8 to 12 minutes or until tender. Peel and mash. Stir cabbage, onion, milk and margarine into mashed potatoes. Place in a 2 L (2-quart) dish. Top with cheese and pepper. Microwave at High for 3 to 4 minutes or until thoroughly reheated. (May be made in advance and reheated.)

MAKES	4 servings
EACH SERVING	375 mL (1-1/2 cups)

1 FRUITS AND VEGETABLES CHOICE	27 g carbohydrates
1 STARCHY CHOICE	6 g protein
1/2 MILK CHOICE	4 g fat
	155 calories

POTATOES AND ONIONS

A different way to serve plain potatoes.

2	medium potatoes, cut in 0.5 cm (1/4-in) slices	2
15 mL	butter OR margarine	1 tbsp
1	medium onion, cut in 0.5 cm (1/4-in) slices	1

Place potatoes in a pie plate or 1.5 L (1.5-quart) casserole. Add butter or margarine. Cover and microwave at High for 3 minutes, stirring halfway through the cooking time. Stir in onion. Cover and microwave at High for 3-1/2 to 4-1/2 minutes. Allow 3 to 5 minutes aftercooking time.

MAKES 4 servings
EACH SERVING 125 mL (1/2 cup)

1 STARCHY CHOICE 18 g carbohydrates
1 EXTRA CHOICE 4 g fat
1 FATS AND OILS CHOICE 113 calories

CREAMY SCALLOPED POTATOES

Sprinkle with a little grated cheese during aftercooking time for an au gratin version.

250 mL	2% milk	1 cup
15 mL	all-purpose flour	1 tbsp
5 mL	cornstarch	1 tsp
	Salt to taste	
5 mL	vegetable oil	1 tsp
	Pepper, thyme, basil, oregano or parsley to taste	
500 g	potatoes	1 lb

In a 1 L (1-quart) measure, combine milk, flour, cornstarch and salt. Whisk until completely mixed. Microwave at High for 2 to 3 minutes, stirring every minute until mixture comes to a boil and thickens. Stir in oil. Season with desired seasonings.

Peel and slice potatoes. Combine potatoes with sauce in a 2 L (2-quart) casserole. Cover and microwave at High for 10 to 15 minutes, stirring twice. Allow 5 minutes aftercooking time, covered.

MAKES	5 servings
EACH SERVING	125 mL (1/2 cup)

1 MILK (2%) CHOICE	21 g carbohydrates
1 STARCHY CHOICE	4 g protein
	2 g fat
	114 calories

SPINACH SPAGHETTI SAUCE

It is often stated that pasta is not fattening, and this is a fact. It is usually the sauce that contains the calories. Try this delicious vegetarian sauce and enjoy pasta often. Cook the pasta in your microwave oven, especially during the summer, to reduce humidity in the kitchen.

1	carrot	1
1	green pepper	1
250 g	fresh spinach	1/2 lb
1	onion	1
750 mL	ground tomatoes	3 cups
15 mL	dried parsley	1 tbsp
5 mL	oregano	1 tsp
5 mL	garlic powder	1 tsp
2 mL	freshly ground pepper	1/2 tsp
250 mL	water	1 cup

Combine all ingredients in a food processor or blender. Purée until vegetables are well chopped. Pour into a 3 L (3-quart) casserole. Cover with tight lid or microwave-safe plastic wrap. Microwave at High for 10 minutes, then at Medium (70%) for 15 to 20 minutes. Serve over pasta.

See p. 123 for instructions on how to cook pasta.

MAKES	4 servings
EACH SERVING	250 mL (1 cup)

1 FRUITS AND VEGETABLES CHOICE	11 g carbohydrates
	2 g protein
	53 calories

TOMATOES WITH PARMESAN CHEESE

A simple, easy and delicious way to use up those fall tomatoes.

....

2	tomatoes	2
10 mL	grated Parmesan cheese	2 tsp
pinch	basil	pinch
	Pepper to taste	

....

Tomatoes should be medium ripe, as very ripe tomatoes will take less time. Halve tomatoes crosswise, keeping portions as equal as possible. Arrange in a round dish with a space between each. Combine cheese, basil and pepper. Sprinkle over tomatoes. Cover and microwave at High power for 1 to 1-1/2 minutes. Rotate each tomato half, cover, and microwave at High for another 1 to 1-1/2 minutes. Allow 2 minutes aftercooking time.

....

MAKES 4 servings
EACH SERVING 1/2 tomato

....

1 EXTRA CHOICE

2 g carbohydrates
1 g protein
12 calories

TURNIP (RUTABAGA)

When I was told I would never again have to cut up a raw turnip, I was intrigued. This easy method was given to me by Marilyn Stewart, a microwave cooking consultant with Panasonic. I love it!

1	turnip or rutabaga, about 500 g (1 lb)	1

Pierce turnip with a fork 5 or 6 times. Place on a paper plate or several layers of paper towels. Microwave at High 22 to 25 minutes per kg (10 to 12 minutes per lb). Allow 10 minutes aftercooking time. Peel by scraping with a butter knife. Cut, mash and serve.

MAKES 6 servings (750 mL/3 cups)
EACH SERVING 125 mL (1/2 cup)

1 FRUITS AND VEGETABLES CHOICE 10 g carbohydrates
1 g protein
44 calories

ZUCCHINI AND TOMATOES

Microwaving vegetables allows for many combinations. This is just one example. Use your imagination for others.

250 mL	zucchini slices, 0.5 cm (1/4-in) thick	1 cup
10 mL	butter OR margarine	2 tsp
250 mL	tomato wedges, 0.5 cm (1/4-in) thick	1 cup

Place zucchini slices in a pie plate or 1.5 L (1.5-quart) casserole. Add butter or margarine. Cover, microwave at High for 2 minutes. Stir in tomato wedges. Cover, microwave at High for 1 to 2-1/2 minutes. Allow 3 to 5 minutes aftercooking time.

1 EXTRA CHOICE	3.5 g carbohydrates
1/2 FATS AND OILS CHOICE	2.5 g fat
	37 calories

JAPANESE VEGETABLES

A family favorite that deserves to be served to company.

1	small zucchini	1
2	stalks celery	2
1	small green pepper	1
2	stalks broccoli	2
3	green onions	3
1	tomato	1
15 mL	salad oil	1 tbsp
15 mL	soya sauce	1 tbsp
1	clove garlic, crushed	1
0.5 mL	ground ginger	1/8 tsp
0.5 mL	dry mustard	1/8 tsp

Slice unpeeled zucchini and celery lengthwise. Core and seed green pepper and cut into small strips. Break broccoli into florets. Cut green onions into small pieces. Combine all vegetables and arrange in a pie plate. Cut tomato into eight wedges and arrange on top of vegetables. In a small bowl, combine salad oil, soya sauce, garlic, ginger and dry mustard. Mix thoroughly. Pour sauce over vegetables. Cover with another pie plate or microwave-safe plastic wrap. Microwave at High for 3 to 4 minutes.

| MAKES | 4 servings |
| EACH SERVING | approximately 175 mL (3/4 cup) |

1 EXTRA CHOICE	3.5 g carbohydrates
1 FATS AND OILS CHOICE	5 g fat
	59 calories

CORN, PEPPER AND ONION STIR FRY

Many of my students thought it was impossible to stir-fry in the micro-wave oven. It can be done easily and often, with fewer calories!

300 mL	frozen corn	1-1/4 cups
15 mL	butter OR margarine	1 tbsp
75 mL	chopped green pepper	1/3 cup
75 mL	sliced green onions	1/3 cup

Place frozen corn in a small casserole and microwave at High for 2 to 3 minutes or until separated. Preheat browning skillet for 2 minutes. Add butter or margarine with corn, green pepper and green onions. Cover and microwave at High for 4-1/2 to 7-1/2 minutes, stirring after half the cooking time. Allow 3 to 5 minutes aftercooking time.

MAKES	4 servings
EACH SERVING	approximately 125 mL (1/2 cup)

1 STARCHY CHOICE	18.5 g carbohydrates
1 EXTRA CHOICE	4 g fat
1 FATS AND OILS CHOICE	127 calories

CARROT AND CELERY STIR FRY

An interesting combination of color and texture.

15 mL	butter OR margarine	1 tbsp
250 mL	carrots, cut in 0.5 cm (1/4-in) slices	1 cup
250 mL	sliced celery	1 cup

Preheat browning skillet for 2 minutes. Add butter or margarine with carrots and celery. Cover and microwave at High for 3-1/2 to 5-1/2 minutes, stirring halfway through cooking time. Allow 3 to 5 minutes aftercooking time.

MAKES	4 servings
EACH SERVING	125 mL (1/2 cup)

1 FRUITS AND VEGETABLES CHOICE	11 g carbohydrates
1 FATS AND OILS CHOICE	4 g fat
	93 calories

BROCCOLI AND CAULIFLOWER STIR FRY

Add a few wedges of tomato or red pepper for more color.

15 mL	butter OR margarine	1 tbsp
325 mL	broccoli florets	1-1/3 cups
325 mL	cauliflower florets	1-1/3 cups
50 mL	sliced almonds	1/4 cup
10 mL	soya sauce	2 tsp

Preheat browning skillet for 2 minutes. Add butter or margarine with remaining ingredients. Cover and microwave at High for 4 to 6-1/2 minutes, stirring halfway through the cooking time. Allow 3 to 5 minutes aftercooking time.

MAKES	4 servings
EACH SERVING	175 mL (3/4 cup)

1 EXTRA CHOICE	3.5 g carbohydrates
1 FATS AND OILS CHOICE	5 g fat
	59 calories

SNOWPEA, MUSHROOM AND BEAN SPROUT STIR FRY

When fresh snowpeas are available, this is a must.

15 mL	butter OR margarine	1 tbsp
20	fresh OR frozen snowpea pods	20
250 mL	fresh mushrooms, cut in 0.5 cm (1/4-in) slices	1 cup
125 mL	bean sprouts, fresh or canned	1/2 cup

Preheat browning skillet for 2 minutes. Add butter or margarine with snowpea pods, mushrooms and bean sprouts. Cover and microwave at High for 3-1/2 to 6-1/2 minutes, stirring halfway through the cooking time. Allow 3 to 5 minutes aftercooking time.

MAKES	4 servings
EACH SERVING	1/4 of recipe with 5 snowpea pods

1/2 FRUITS AND VEGETABLES CHOICE	13.5 g carbohydrates
1 EXTRA CHOICE	5 g fat
1 FATS AND OILS CHOICE	81 calories

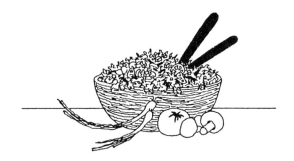

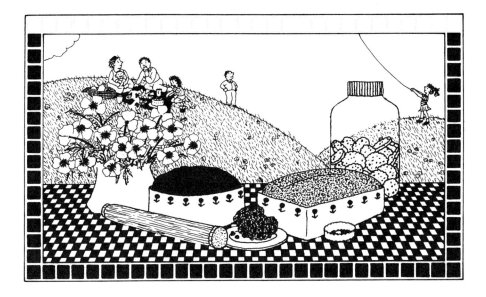

Baking can be very successful when carried out with the help of your microwave oven. Keep the following tips in mind:

- Let batter stand 10 to 15 minutes before baking. This allows the leavening agents to begin the rising process, resulting in lighter, fluffier baked goods.
- If using a conventional recipe, mix the ingredients in the same quantities and manner. Follow the Quick Reference Chart for approximate cooking times and powers.
- Remove baked goods when the surface appears damp—if touched, it would come off on your hand. Allow 10 to 15 minutes aftercooking time.
- If bottom surface of baked good is wet, line utensil with paper towel the next time you bake it.

  Muffins use a small quantity of batter and thus become more difficult to bake in a microwave oven. Some steps that will increase your success are:

- Combine wet and dry ingredients until just moistened. Beating until smooth toughens muffins.
- If using a conventional recipe, mix ingredients in the same quantities and manner. Follow the Quick Reference Chart for approximate cooking times and powers.
- Let batter stand 10 to 15 minutes before baking. This allows the leavening agents to begin the rising process, resulting in lighter, fluffier baked goods.

- Line the microwave-safe muffin utensil with one or two muffin papers. This will help absorb excess moisture.
- Fill each cup two-thirds full—about 25 mL (2 tbsp) of batter.

Scratch bread recipes and frozen unbaked loaves can be proofed and baked in your microwave oven. Place the dough in a greased loaf pan. Place 250 mL (1 cup) water in a microwave-safe measuring cup and set in oven next to the loaf pan. Cover both water and dough with one cover. Microwave at Warm (10%) for 20 to 25 minutes. Dough will double in this time. *Do not punch down*! The yeast is killed during this one-stage proofing. Bake at Medium (70%) for 10 to 11 minutes per loaf. To brown the top of the bread, brush with egg white, milk, or water and sprinkle with bran, cornmeal or wheat germ. If the bread is savoury, brush with soya sauce, Worcestershire sauce or bouillon and top with chopped onions, grated cheese or sesame seeds.

QUICK REFERENCE CHART
BAKED GOODS

TYPE	QUANTITY OF BATTER	DISH	POWER (may be 2-step)	TIME
BUTTER CAKE	625 mL (2-1/2 cups)	20-23 cm (8-9 in) round or square	Low (30%) High	6 min. 2 to 5 min.
BROWN-IES	500 mL (2 cups)	same	Med-Low (50%)	9 to 11 min.
MUFFINS AND CUP-CAKES	[15 mL (2 tbsp)] × 6	6-cup muffin utensil	High OR Medium (70%)	2 to 2-1/2 min. 3 to 5 min.
BREAD	1 loaf	glass loaf pan	Medium (70%)	10 to 11 min.

FERGOSA BREAD

This recipe came from my friend Joan, who told me it was super. I converted it to microwave cooking with very tasty results.

125 mL	chopped onion	1/2 cup
75 mL	milk	1/3 cup
15 mL	margarine	1 tbsp
250 mL	grated cheese	1 cup
250 mL	biscuit mix	1 cup
1	egg	1
	Poppy seeds	

In a 22 cm (9-in) pie plate, combine onion, milk and margarine. Microwave at High for 2 to 3 minutes or until onion is transparent. Stir in grated cheese, biscuit mix and egg. Toss with a fork until ingredients are just combined. Top with poppy seeds. Microwave at Medium (70%) for 6 to 6-1/2 minutes. Bread will be moist on top. Allow 5 minutes aftercooking time. Serve warm or cold.

| MAKES | 8 servings |
| EACH SERVING | 1/8 of loaf |

1 PROTEIN CHOICE	11.5 g carbohydrates
1 FRUITS AND VEGETABLES CHOICE	6.5 g protein
1 FATS AND OILS CHOICE	9 g fat
	150 calories

APPLESAUCE-OAT BREAD

This grainy, moist cake is wonderful with coffee or tea. Try topping it with the Strawberry Jam or Apple Jelly featured in this book (pp. 213 and 212).

250 mL	whole wheat flour	1 cup
250 mL	all-purpose flour	1 cup
250 mL	rolled oats	1 cup
20 mL	baking powder	4 tsp
2 mL	cinnamon	1/2 tsp
2 mL	nutmeg	1/2 tsp
1 mL	allspice	1/4 tsp
1 mL	baking soda	1/4 tsp
1	egg, beaten	1
250 mL	unsweetened applesauce	1 cup
125 mL	water	1/2 cup
15 mL	oil	1 tbsp

In a large bowl, combine flours, oats, baking powder, cinnamon, nutmeg, allspice and baking soda. Mix well. In a separate bowl, combine egg, applesauce, water and oil. Pour liquids into dry ingredients and stir until well combined. Pour batter into a ring mould pan. Microwave at Low (30%) for 6 minutes, then at High for 5 to 6 minutes. Allow 10 minutes aftercooking time and turn out of pan.

MAKES	16 slices
EACH SERVING	1 slice

1 STARCHY CHOICE	18 g carbohydrates
1 FATS AND OILS CHOICE	3 g protein
1 EXTRA CHOICE	4 g fat
	96 calories

BLUEBERRY MUFFINS

Do you need a muffin utensil for the microwave oven? Not necessarily. Try lining microwave-safe tea mugs, coffee cups or custard cups with muffin papers. Don't give up on cooking certain recipes because you don't own the proper utensil—experiment and enjoy all the foods you love.

375 mL	all-purpose flour	1-1/2 cups
15 mL	baking powder	1 tbsp
2 mL	cinnamon	1/2 tsp
2 mL	nutmeg	1/2 tsp
2	eggs, beaten	2
50 mL	vegetable oil	1/4 cup
175 mL	orange juice	3/4 cup
5 mL	grated lemon peel	1 tsp
250 mL	blueberries (See note)	1 cup

In a large bowl, combine flour, baking powder, cinnamon and nutmeg. In a separate bowl, combine eggs, oil, juice, and lemon peel. Pour into dry ingredients and toss with fork just until combined. Stir in blueberries.

Line a microwave-safe muffin utensil with double muffin papers. Fill each paper with 25 mL (2 tbsp) batter. Microwave at High for 2 to 2-1/2 minutes for 6 muffins. Allow 5 minutes aftercooking time.

Note: Blueberries may be frozen or fresh. If frozen, toss with 10 mL (2 tsp) flour before combining with butter.

MAKES	12 muffins
EACH SERVING	1 muffin

1 STARCHY CHOICE	16 g carbohydrates
1 FATS AND OILS CHOICE	3 g protein
	6 g fat
	130 calories

OATMEAL RAISIN MUFFINS

This recipe is my all-time favorite. It was given to me at Peterborough Civic Hospital when I was in for the birth of my second daughter. I changed the recipe to suit microwave cooking.

250 mL	buttermilk	1 cup
250 mL	rolled oats	1 cup
125 mL	raisins	1/2 cup
250 mL	whole wheat flour	1 cup
5 mL	baking powder	1 tsp
2 mL	baking soda	1/2 tsp
25 mL	wheat germ	2 tbsp
75 mL	vegetable oil	1/3 cup
15 mL	honey	1 tbsp
1	egg, beaten	1

In a small bowl, combine buttermilk, oats and raisins. Microwave at High for 1-1/2 minutes or until buttermilk is hot. Let stand 10 minutes. In a large bowl, combine flour, baking powder, baking soda and wheat germ. Stir in oil, honey and egg. Add oat mixture. Stir with fork until just combined.

Line a microwave-safe muffin utensil with double muffin papers. Fill each paper with 25 mL (2 tbsp) batter. Microwave at High for 2 to 2-1/2 minutes for 6 muffins. Allow 5 minutes aftercooking time.

MAKES	18 muffins
EACH SERVING	1 muffin

1 FRUITS AND VEGETABLES CHOICE	10 g carbohydrates
1/2 FATS AND OILS CHOICE	2.5 g protein
	1.2 g fat
	95 calories

BRAN MUFFINS

Muffins will appear moist on the top when taken from the microwave oven. Allow full aftercooking time for the muffins to finish cooking and moistness to disappear.

250 mL	all-purpose flour	1 cup
250 mL	bran	1 cup
75 mL	lightly packed brown sugar	1/3 cup
15 mL	baking powder	1 tbsp
2 mL	cinnamon	1/2 tsp
2 mL	nutmeg	1/2tsp
	Salt to taste	
250 mL	2% milk	1 cup
50 mL	vegetable oil	1/4 cup
1	egg	1

In a large mixing bowl, combine flour, bran, brown sugar, baking powder, cinnamon, nutmeg and salt. Combine milk, oil and egg and beat lightly. Add milk mixture to dry ingredients and stir just enough to mix; do not beat. Batter will appear lumpy.

Fill microwave-safe muffin utensil or custard cups lined with double paper liners 2/3 full. Microwave at Medium (70%) for 4 to 5 minutes for 6 muffins. Allow 5 minutes aftercooking time.

MAKES	12 muffins
EACH SERVING	1 muffin

1 STARCHY CHOICE	14 g carbohydrates
1 FATS AND OILS CHOICE	3 g protein
	6 g fat
	122 calories

DATE-NUT BRAN MUFFINS

My favorite. In only 5 minutes I can enjoy a hot muffin.

250 mL	all-purpose flour	1 cup
250 mL	bran	1 cup
75 mL	lightly packed brown sugar	1/3 cup
15 mL	baking powder	1 tbsp
2 mL	cinnamon	1/2 tsp
2 mL	nutmeg	1/2 tsp
2 mL	allspice	1/2 tsp
	Salt to taste	
125 mL	chopped dates	1/2 cup
50 mL	chopped nuts	1/4 cup
250 mL	2% milk	1 cup
50 mL	vegetable oil	1/4 cup
1	egg	1

In a large mixing bowl, combine flour, bran, brown sugar, baking powder, spices, salt, dates and nuts. Combine milk, oil and egg and beat lightly. Add milk mixture to dry ingredients and stir just enough to mix; do not beat. Batter will appear lumpy.

Fill microwave-safe muffin utensil or custard cups lined with double paper liners 2/3 full. Microwave at Medium (70%) for 4 to 5 minutes for 6 muffins. Allow 5 minutes aftercooking time.

Note: Muffins will appear moist on the top; this will disappear while standing.

MAKES	12 muffins
EACH SERVING	1 muffin

1 STARCHY CHOICE	24 g carbohydrates
1 FRUITS AND VEGETABLES CHOICE	4 g protein
1 FATS AND OILS CHOICE	6 g fat
	166 calories

BUTTERMILK OAT BRAN MUFFINS

Muffins will not brown in the microwave oven, but do cook up nice and fluffy. Let the batter stand 10 minutes or so before cooking to let the leavening agents begin to work.

250 mL	oat bran	1 cup
250 mL	whole wheat flour	1 cup
250 mL	all-purpose flour	1 cup
10 mL	baking powder	2 tsp
2 mL	baking soda	1/2 tsp
1	egg, beaten	1
25 mL	vegetable oil	2 tbsp
50 mL	molasses	1/4 cup
375 mL	buttermilk	1-1/2 cups

In a large bowl, combine oat bran, flours, baking powder and baking soda. In a separate bowl, combine egg, oil, molasses and buttermilk. Stir into dry ingredients.

Line a microwave-safe muffin utensil with double muffin papers. Fill each paper 2/3 full. Microwave at High for 2 to 2-1/2 minutes for 6 muffins. Allow 5 minutes aftercooking time.

MAKES	18 muffins
EACH SERVING	1 muffin

1-1/2 STARCHY CHOICES	26 g carbohydrates
1/2 MILK CHOICE	5.5 g protein
	8 g fat
	160 calories

WHEAT AND WALNUT MUFFINS

Hearty and healthy are two words this recipe brings to mind. Walnuts with wheat germ make a tasty couple in these easy-to-prepare muffins. All the ingredients can be easily kept on hand to be available any time.

375 mL	all-purpose flour	1-1/2 cups
10 mL	baking powder	2 tsp
25 mL	wheat germ	2 tbsp
1	egg, beaten	1
250 mL	skim milk	1 cup
250 mL	chopped walnuts	1 cup

In a large bowl, combine flour, baking powder and wheat germ. In a separate bowl, combine egg and milk. Pour milk into dry ingredients. Toss with a fork until just combined. Stir in walnuts.

Line a microwave-safe muffin utensil with double muffin papers. Fill each paper with 25 mL (2 tbsp) batter. Microwave at High for 2 to 2-1/2 minutes. Allow 5 minutes aftercooking time.

MAKES	12 muffins
EACH SERVING	1 muffin

1 STARCHY CHOICE	15 g carbohydrates
1/2 PROTEIN CHOICE	4.5 g protein
1/2 FATS AND OILS CHOICE	6 g fat
	134 calories

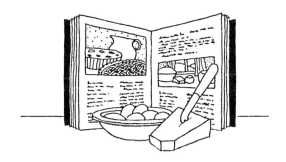

PUMPKIN MUFFINS

Muffin mania is still with us, and you can join the craze! Enjoy these muffins as snacks or for breakfast and lunch Starchy choices. Muffins are so fast to prepare in your microwave oven.

250 mL	bran	1 cup
250 mL	all-purpose flour	1 cup
125 mL	bulk sweetener	1/2 cup
5 mL	cinnamon	1 tsp
5 mL	baking powder	1 tsp
5 mL	baking soda	1 tsp
2 mL	salt	1/2 tsp
250 mL	canned pumpkin	1 cup
1	egg, slightly beaten	1
75 mL	vegetable oil	1/3 cup
125 mL	skim milk	1/2 cup
250 mL	raisins	1 cup

In a large bowl, combine bran, flour, sweetener, cinnamon, baking powder, baking soda and salt. Combine pumpkin, egg, oil and milk. Stir into dry ingredients. Stir in raisins.

Place medium muffin papers in vented microwave-safe muffin utensil. Fill 6 muffin papers with 50 mL (1/4 cup) batter. Microwave at High for 2 to 2-1/2 minutes. Allow 5 minutes aftercooking time.

MAKES	24 muffins
EACH SERVING	1 muffin

1/2 STARCHY CHOICE	10 g carbohydrates
1/2 FATS AND OILS CHOICE	1.5 g protein
1 EXTRA CHOICE	3 g fat
	70 calories

MICROWAVED CHOCOLATE CHIP COOKIES

Our cookie jar is always filled with these yummy treats.

125 mL	butter OR margarine	1/2 cup
50 mL	lightly packed brown sugar	1/4 cup
1	egg	1
10 mL	vanilla	2 tsp
250 mL	all-purpose flour	1 cup
2 mL	baking soda	1/2 tsp
2 mL	cinnamon	1/2 tsp
	Salt to taste	
125 mL	rolled oats	1/2 cup
125 mL	semi-sweet chocolate chips	1/2 cup

Cream butter or margarine with sugar until light and fluffy. Beat in egg and vanilla. In a separate bowl, combine flour, baking soda, cinnamon and salt. Stir into creamed mixture. Fold in oats and chocolate chips. Drop 10 mL (2 tsp) batter onto microwave-safe cookie pan or large plate. Microwave at Medium (70%) for 2-1/2 minutes for 12 cookies.

MAKES 48 cookies

EACH SERVING 2 cookies

1 FRUITS AND VEGETABLES CHOICE

1 FATS AND OILS CHOICE

10 g carbohydrates

1 g protein

6 g fat

98 calories

MICROWAVED PEANUT BUTTER COOKIES

Cookies can be successfully baked in a microwave oven. This recipe will satisfy the "Cookie Monster" in all of us.

375 mL	triticale flour (See note)	1-1/2 cups
5 mL	baking powder	1 tsp
2 mL	salt	1/2 tsp
50 mL	margarine	1/4 cup
125 mL	smooth peanut butter	1/2 cup
5 mL	vanilla	1 tsp
1	egg, beaten	1
75 mL	orange juice	1/3 cup
125 mL	bulk sweetener	1/2 cup

In a medium mixing bowl or food processor, combine flour, baking powder and salt. In a measuring cup, combine margarine, peanut butter, vanilla, egg and orange juice. Add liquids to dry ingredients. Mix until combined. Add sweetener. Stir. Measure 15 mL (1 tbsp) dough for each cookie. Place 6 cookies on a microwave-safe dinner plate. Flatten with a fork. Microwave at High for 1 minute and 15 seconds. Repeat until all dough is used.

MAKES	48 cookies
EACH SERVING	1 cookie

1/2 FRUITS AND VEGETABLES CHOICE	5 g carbohydrates
1 FATS AND OILS CHOICE	2.5 g protein
	5 g fat
	75 calories

Note: Triticale flour is made from rye, wheat and oats. It's available at bulk food stores. Can be replaced with all-purpose flour.

SHORTBREAD

A Christmas treat that deserves to be served year round.

250 g	butter at room temperature	1/2 lb
125 mL	sugar	1/2 cup
125 mL	rice flour	1/2 cup
425 mL	all-purpose flour	1-3/4 cups

Cream butter with sugar until fluffy. Stir in flours until well blended. Roll out onto lightly floured surface to 6 mm (1/4-in) thickness. Using 4 cm (1-1/2 in) round cookie cutter, cut out cookies. Place 12 cookies, evenly spaced, on microwave-safe pan or plate. Microwave at Medium (70%) for 2 to 3 minutes. Do not allow to brown. Undercook the first batch, then microwave for 10-second intervals until desired doneness is achieved.

Note: If browning occurs, reduce cooking time by 10 seconds.

MAKES	60 cookies
EACH SERVING	2 cookies

1 FRUITS AND VEGETABLES CHOICE	10 g carbohydrates
1-1/2 FATS AND OILS CHOICES	8 g fat
	112 calories

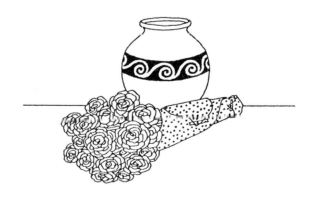

IRISH SCONES

Scratch baking in your microwave oven can give excellent results. Try these Irish Scones with a stew or chili meal.

75 mL	margarine	1/3 cup
500 mL	flour	2 cups
5 mL	baking soda	1 tsp
5 mL	cream of tartar	1 tsp
pinch	salt	pinch
50 mL	currants	1/4 cup
25 mL	sugar	2 tbsp
125 mL	water	1/2 cup
125 mL	plain yogurt	1/2 cup
50 mL	flour	1/4 cup
	Cinnamon to taste	

In a mixing bowl, cream together margarine, flour, baking soda, cream of tartar and salt. Stir in currants and sugar. In a separate bowl, combine water and yogurt. Pour yogurt mix onto dry ingredients. Using 50 mL (1/4 cup) flour, roll out dough until 1 cm (1/2-in) thick. Cut into 24 rounds using a biscuit cutter or glass. Sprinkle each scone with cinnamon. Arrange 6 scones on a microwave-safe dinner plate and microwave at Medium (70%) for 2 to 2-1/2 minutes or until dry to the touch. Repeat until all rounds are baked.

MAKES	24 scones
EACH SERVING	1 scone

1 FATS AND OILS CHOICE	11 g carbohydrates
1/2 STARCHY CHOICE	1.7 g protein
1/2 MILK CHOICE	6 g fat
	76 calories

GRAHAM CRACKER CRUST

You will find many uses for this versatile crust. Start with Lemon Chiffon Pie (p. 209) or Pumpkin Light Pie (p. 210).

....

50 mL	butter OR margarine	3 tbsp
175 mL	graham wafer crumbs	3/4 cup
1 mL	cinnamon	1/4 tsp
1 mL	nutmeg	1/4 tsp
0.5 mL	allspice	1/8 tsp

....

Melt butter or margarine in a pie plate at High for 30 to 45 seconds. Combine graham wafer crumbs, cinnamon, nutmeg and allspice. Add to pie plate and combine well with a fork. Spread evenly over bottom of pie plate. Microwave at High for 3 to 5 minutes, watching carefully to prevent scorching. Allow to cool before filling.

....

| **MAKES** | 1 pie crust, 8 wedges |
| **EACH SERVING** | 1 wedge (crust only) |

....

1/2 STARCHY CHOICE	7 g carbohydrates
1 FATS AND OILS CHOICE	1 g protein
	5 g fat
	77 calories

OATMEAL CRUST

A change in taste from the graham pie crust. Try with Chocolate Pie (p. 208).

....

175 mL	all-purpose flour	3/4 cup
125 mL	rolled oats	1/2 cup
1 mL	cinnamon	1/4 tsp
	Salt to taste	
50 mL	vegetable oil	1/4 cup
45 to 50 mL	ice water	3 to 4 tbsp

....

Combine flour, rolled oats, cinnamon and salt in a mixing bowl. Slowly drizzle in oil, mixing with a fork, until mixture resembles fine crumbs. Add ice water a few drops at a time until mixture starts to form a ball. Press into 22 cm (9-in) pie plate. Microwave at High for 4 to 6 minutes, watching carefully to prevent scorching. Allow to cool before filling.

MAKES	1 pie crust, 6 wedges	
EACH SERVING	1 wedge (crust only)	

1 STARCHY CHOICE	15 g carbohydrates
2 FATS AND OILS CHOICES	3 g protein
	10 g fat
	162 calories

WALNUT OATMEAL CRUST

This different pie crust is terrific filled with Chocolate Pie (p. 208) or Butterscotch Pie (p. 207).

75 mL	margarine	1/3 cup
250 mL	rolled oats	1 cup
175 mL	crushed walnuts	3/4 cup

In a 22 cm (9-in) microwave-safe pie plate, melt margarine at High for 30 to 45 seconds. Add oats and spread out evenly. Microwave at High for 2 to 3 minutes or until oats begin to turn golden brown. Stir. Add walnuts. Press mixture onto sides of pie plate. Microwave at High for 1 minute and allow to cool before filling.

MAKES	1 pie crust, 8 wedges	
EACH SERVING	1 wedge (crust only)	

3 FATS AND OILS CHOICES	5 g carbohydrates
1/2 FRUITS AND VEGETABLES CHOICE	1.4 g protein
	14 g fat
	161 calories

CINNAMON COFFEE CAKE

Have your cake and eat it too! Just because we follow a diabetic choice diet doesn't mean we are deprived. This light cake is wonderful with morning coffee or at tea time.

250 mL	plain yogurt	1 cup
5 mL	baking soda	1 tsp
50 mL	margarine	1/4 cup
1	egg	1
	Sweetener equivalent to	
	125 mL (1/2 cup) sugar	
5 mL	vanilla	1 tsp
375 mL	flour	1-1/2 cups
10 mL	baking powder	2 tsp
15 mL	cinnamon	1 tbsp
10 mL	nutmeg	2 tsp
2 mL	ground cloves	1/2 tsp

In a mixing bowl, combine yogurt and baking soda. Let stand 5 minutes. Cream margarine and egg into yogurt mixture. Add vanilla. In a separate bowl, combine flour and baking powder. Add dry ingredients to wet and stir until just combined. Combine cinnamon, nutmeg and cloves. Sprinkle half of cinnamon mixture into a 22 cm (9-in) square dish. Pour in half of batter and repeat. Microwave at Low (30%) for 6 minutes, then at High for 2-1/2 to 3 minutes. Allow 5 minutes aftercooking time. Turn out of dish and serve warm or cool.

MAKES	12 slices
EACH SERVING	1 slice

1 STARCHY CHOICE	14 g carbohydrates
1 FATS AND OILS CHOICE	3 g protein
	6 g fat
	121 calories

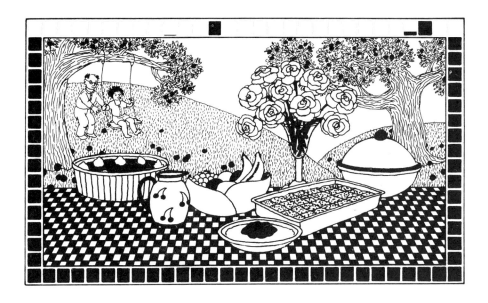

Desserts add the finishing touches to a meal; they can be simple or dazzling. Almost everyone enjoys desserts, and people with diabetes are no exception. The desserts in this section help the person with diabetes to adhere to the meal plan as well as satisfy the sweet tooth. Choose an appropriate dessert: not only should it contrast the main course of the meal, but for a person with diabetes, the dessert must suit the meal requirements. A person with diabetes should make note of the food choices allowed for a meal and then choose a dessert to fill out the requirements or plan the meal around the dessert choice. For example, Pumpkin Light Pie would be an acceptable choice to round out a light meal.

Sugar is used in some of the recipes; this is a controlled amount and has been included in the carbohydrates and food choice values. Sugar is available in many forms, such as white and brown sugar, honey, syrup, molasses, and most ingredients ending in "ose." Natural sugars are found in fruits, vegetables, juices and milk; the acceptable amounts of these foods are listed in your Good Health Eating Guide.

The key factor in how the body digests sugar is the amount consumed. Natural sugars and added sugars in the form of white or brown sugar, honey, syrups, molasses and so on will raise the blood sugar level quickly. For this reason, you should consume natural sugars as well as added sugars in controlled amounts.

Making desserts in the microwave oven is fast and easy. Sometimes it may be a good idea to prepare a diabetic dessert as well as a sugar-laden "non-diabetic" dessert for the other family members. If time does not permit the preparation of two desserts, certainly the entire family can benefit from the diabetic dessert, which is in any case healthier, since it contains less added sugar.

Fruits are ideal prepared in the microwave oven. During the winter months, warmed fruit with a dash of spices is a welcome treat. Avoid overcooking; usually slight heating is all that is required. Fresh microwaved fruits are best served tender-crisp. Covering the fruit allows it to cook more evenly. Frozen fruit will defrost quickly and easily at High power. Stir frequently to separate, but be careful not to overdefrost and begin cooking. A 300 mL (10 oz) package of frozen fruit will require 1 to 2 minutes at High, covered. Let aftercook for 5 minutes, then separate with a fork. Fruit should still have ice crystals, but only needs a few minutes to completely defrost before it can be served.

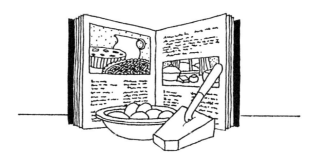

APPLESAUCE

Almond flavoring adds pizzazz!

1 kg	apples	2 lb
25 mL	lemon juice	2 tbsp
125 mL	water	1/2 cup
1 mL	cinnamon	1/4 tsp
1 - 2 drops	almond flavoring (optional)	1 - 2 drops
	Sweetener to taste	

Peel, core and slice apples into equal bite-size pieces. Measure 1.5 L (6 cups) into a 4 L (4-quart) casserole with lemon juice and water. Cover and microwave at High for 9 to 10 minutes, stirring 2 or 3 times, until apples are soft. Allow 4 to 5 minutes aftercooking time. Add cinnamon, almond flavoring and sweetener. Mash with a wooden spoon, or purée if desired.

MAKES   10 servings
EACH SERVING   75 mL (1/3 cup)

1 FRUITS AND VEGETABLES CHOICE   10 g carbohydrates
                                            40 calories

APPLE CRISP

Substitute peaches or pears when they are in season.

1 L	apples, peeled, cored and sliced	4 cups
15 mL	lemon juice	1 tbsp
25 mL	butter OR margarine	2 tbsp
175 mL	rolled oats	3/4 cup
25 mL	brown sugar	2 tbsp
25 mL	chopped nuts	2 tbsp
1 mL	cinnamon	1/4 tsp

Place apples in a microwave baking pan and sprinkle with lemon juice. In a small bowl, melt butter or margarine at High for 30 to 45 seconds. Stir in rolled oats, brown sugar, nuts and cinnamon. Combine well. Sprinkle evenly over apples. Microwave at High for 8 to 10 minutes. Allow 5 to 7 minutes aftercooking time.

| MAKES | 8 servings |
| EACH SERVING | 125 mL (1/2 cup) |

1 FRUITS AND VEGETABLES CHOICE	10 g carbohydrates
1 FATS AND OILS CHOICE	1 g protein
	5 g fat
	89 calories

APPLE GINGERBREAD

A special treat for a special occasion!

5 to 6	apples	5 to 6
50 mL	shortening	1/4 cup
50 mL	lightly packed brown sugar	1/4 cup
75 mL	molasses	1/3 cup
1	egg	1
375 mL	all-purpose flour	1-1/2 cups
5 mL	salt	1 tsp
5 mL	baking soda	1 tsp
5 mL	cinnamon	1 tsp
5 mL	ground ginger	1 tsp
1 mL	ground cloves	1/4 tsp
175 mL	boiling water	3/4 cup

Peel, core and slice apples and arrange in a pie plate. In a large bowl cream shortening with sugar until light and fluffy. Beat in molasses and egg. In a separate bowl, combine flour, salt, baking soda, cinnamon, ginger and cloves. Stir dry ingredients into creamed mixture alternately with boiling water until just mixed, beginning and ending with dry ingredients. Spoon batter on top of apples. Microwave at Low (30%) for 6 to 7 minutes. Increase power to High and microwave 3 to 4 minutes. Allow 5 to 10 minutes aftercooking time.

MAKES	12 servings
EACH SERVING	1/12 wedge

1/2 STARCHY CHOICE	30 g carbohydrates
2 FRUITS AND VEGETABLES CHOICES	3 g protein
1 FATS AND OILS CHOICE	5 g fat
	177 calories

Note: If you find your oven has difficulties completely cooking the centre in some recipes, insert a glass tumbler, open end up, in the centre of your pie plate.

MINT BLUEBERRIES AND PEACHES

These two fruits can be purchased frozen or fresh and are available all year long. If your exchanges allow, serve this over ice cream or a plain cake for an incredible treat.

2	peaches, peeled	2
125 mL	blueberries	1/2 cup
15 mL	lemon juice	1 tbsp
5 mL	dried mint	1 tsp

Cut peaches into halves. In a 1 L (1-quart) measure, combine all ingredients. Microwave at High for 3 to 4 minutes or until thoroughly warmed.

MAKES 4 servings

EACH SERVING 1/2 peach plus 25 mL (2 tbsp) blueberries and sauce

1 FRUITS AND VEGETABLES CHOICE
8 g carbohydrates
1.5 g protein
31 calories

RUM ORANGES

Fruit desserts offer a wide range of flavor combinations. This couple is a perfectly suited marriage of colors. It is so simple to prepare, yet would be great for a dinner party.

2	oranges, peeled	2
15 mL	chopped dates	1 tbsp
5 mL	rum extract	1 tsp

Slice oranges. In a 500 mL (2-cup) measure, combine all ingredients and microwave at High for 2 to 3 minutes or until thoroughly warmed. Stir.

. . . .

| MAKES | 4 servings |
| EACH SERVING | 125 mL (1/2 cup) |

. . . .

1 FRUITS AND VEGETABLES CHOICE

11.5 g carbohydrates

1 g protein

46 calories

POACHED PEACHES

Try different fruits and combinations of fruits for variety.

. . . .

500 mL	juice from canned peaches, water added	2 cups
5	unsweetened canned peach halves	5
25 mL	lemon juice	2 tbsp
5 mL	vanilla	1 tsp
5 mL	pure orange flavor	1 tsp
	Artificial sweetener to taste	

. . . .

Pour peach juice into measure and add water to make 500 mL (2 cups). Combine peaches, peach juice and lemon juice in a 2 L (2-quart) casserole. Microwave at High for 6 to 8 minutes or until boiling. Add vanilla, orange flavor and sweetener. Allow 5 minutes aftercooking time. Serve warm or cold.

. . . .

| MAKES | 5 servings |
| EACH SERVING | 2 peach halves plus 50 mL (1/4 cup) juice |

. . . .

1 FRUITS AND VEGETABLES CHOICE

10 g carbohydrates

44 calories

SPICED POACHED PEARS

Beautifully colored and delightfully flavored, Spiced Poached Pears are my favorite fruit dessert. I prefer to use fresh Bosc pears, but in the winter, canned pears do nicely.

2	pears, peeled	2
125 mL	cranberry juice	1/2 cup
1 mL	cinnamon	1/4 tsp
2 mL	nutmeg	1/2 tsp
	Grated lemon rind	

Slice pears. Combine all ingredients in a 500 mL (2-cup) measure. Microwave at High for 3 to 4 minutes. Stir and allow 3 minutes aftercooking time. Serve warm.

MAKES	4 servings
EACH SERVING	1/2 pear plus 25 mL (2 tbsp) juice

1-1/2 FRUITS AND VEGETABLES CHOICES	17 g carbohydrates
	.5 g protein
1 EXTRA CHOICE	70 calories

RASPBERRY CHOCOLATE MOUSSE

A wonderful combination of flavors.

50 mL	diet raspberry spread	1/4 cup
2 mL	plain gelatin	1/2 tsp
30 g	grated semi-sweet chocolate	1 oz
2	eggs, separated	2
	Artificial sweetener to taste	

Place diet spread in a small casserole, pressing out into a thin layer. Sprinkle gelatin on top. Microwave at Medium Low (50%) for 2 to 4 minutes, stirring frequently, until gelatin melts and mixture is smooth and starting to boil. Add grated chocolate and stir until smooth. Beat egg yolks. Add to chocolate mixture and blend until smooth. Mixture should thicken slightly; if not, then microwave at Medium Low (50%) for 30-second intervals, being careful not to overcook. Stir in sweetener.

In a medium bowl, beat egg whites until stiff. Combine about 1/4 of egg whites into chocolate mixture. Gently fold chocolate mixture into remaining egg whites. Pour into serving dishes and refrigerate.

MAKES	4 servings
EACH SERVING	75 mL (1/3 cup)

1/2 STARCHY CHOICE	7 g carbohydrates
1/2 PROTEIN CHOICE	5 g protein
1/2 FATS AND OILS CHOICE	3.5 g fat
	85 calories

RHUBARB SAUCE

A spring treat!

500 g	fresh OR frozen rhubarb	1 lb
25 mL	water	2 tbsp
1 - 2 drops	almond flavoring (optional)	1 - 2 drops
	Artificial sweetener to taste	

Cut rhubarb into 2.5 cm (1-in) pieces. Measure 1 L (1 quart) into a 2 L (2-quart) casserole. Cover and microwave at High for 9 to 10 minutes until rhubarb is tender, stirring 2 to 3 times. Allow 4 to 5 minutes aftercooking time. Add almond flavoring and sweetener, and mix well with a wooden spoon. Taste and adjust amount of sweetener according to how sour the rhubarb is.

MAKES	4 servings
EACH SERVING	125 mL (1/2 cup)

1/2 FRUITS AND VEGETABLES CHOICE	4 g carbohydrates
	16 calories

STRAWBERRY SHORTCAKE

What is strawberry season without Strawberry Shortcake? Use your microwave oven for the cake and don't heat up the kitchen! It will be so refreshing after picking (or picking up) those berries.

250 mL	all-purpose flour	1 cup
10 mL	baking powder	2 tsp
1 mL	salt	1/4 tsp
15 mL	bulk sweetener	1 tbsp
50 mL	vegetable oil	3 tbsp
125 mL	skim milk	1/2 cup
500 mL	fresh or frozen strawberries	2 cups
125 mL	plain yogurt	1/2 cup

In a mixing bowl, combine flour, baking powder, salt and sweetener. Add oil and milk. Toss with a fork just until mixture is combined. Using 75 mL (1/3 cup) batter, place 6 shortcakes on a microwave-safe dinner plate. Microwave at Medium (70%) for 3 to 4 minutes or until soft but dry to the touch. Top each shortcake with 75 mL (1/3 cup) strawberries and 15 mL (1 tbsp) yogurt.

MAKES	6 servings
EACH SERVING	1 biscuit plus 75 mL (1/3 cup) berries with 15 mL (1 tbsp) yogurt

1 MILK CHOICE	20 g carbohydrates
1 FATS AND OILS CHOICE	4 g protein
1/2 FRUITS AND VEGETABLES CHOICE	8 g fat
1/2 STARCHY CHOICE	166 calories

FRUIT FLAN

This light dessert is perfect to prepare all year round. Use available seasonal fruits. Combine three, four or more varieties for beautiful results.

250 mL	whole-wheat flour	1 cup
50 mL	cornstarch	1/4 cup
50 mL	bulk sweetener	1/4 cup
75 mL	margarine	1/3 cup
2	egg whites	2
250 mL	cream cheese	1 cup
5 mL	almond extract	1 tsp
500 mL	sliced fresh fruits	2 cups

In a medium mixing bowl, combine flour, cornstarch and sweetener. Cut in margarine with two knives or pastry blender. Stir in egg whites and work to form dough into a ball. Spread dough out onto a 25 cm (10-in) glass serving plate or a 25 cm (10-in) round of cardboard covered with waxed paper. Bake dough at High for 4 to 5 minutes or until crisp.

Combine cream cheese and almond extract in a small bowl. Spread mixture onto crust. Top with sliced fruits. Refrigerate until serving.

MAKES	12 servings
EACH SERVING	1/12 wedge

2 FATS AND OILS CHOICES	15.7 g carbohydrates
1 FRUITS AND VEGETABLES CHOICE	3 g protein
1/2 STARCHY CHOICE	12 g fat
	185 calories

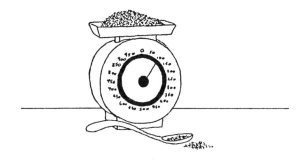

CHOCOLATE MOUSSE DELIGHT

A delightfully light dessert after a full course meal.

1 pkg	plain gelatin	1 pkg
375 mL	skim milk	1-1/2 cups
50 mL	unsweetened cocoa powder	1/4 cup
15 mL	cornstarch	1 tbsp
1	egg, separated	1
	Artificial sweetener equivalent to 125 mL (1/2 cup) sugar	
5 mL	vanilla	1 tsp
50 mL	instant skim milk powder	1/4 cup
50 mL	ice water	1/4 cup

Sprinkle gelatin over 50 mL (1/4 cup) milk to soften. Let stand 5 minutes. In a 2 L (2-quart) measure or bowl, whisk 250 mL (1 cup) milk with cocoa until well mixed. Microwave at Medium Low (50%) for 3 to 5 minutes or until boiling. Reduce power to Low (30%) and microwave for 5 minutes. Combine cornstarch, egg yolk and 50 mL (1/4 cup) milk and stir into cocoa mixture. Microwave at Medium Low (50%) for 1-1/2 to 2 minutes or until mixture thickens. Mix in gelatin and sweetener, stirring until dissolved. Stir in vanilla. Refrigerate until partially set. Combine egg white, skim milk powder and ice water and beat until stiff peaks form. Fold into chocolate mixture. Pour into 6 serving dishes. Refrigerate 4 hours before serving.

MAKES   6 servings
EACH SERVING   approximately 125 mL (1/2 cup)

1 MILK CHOICE

7 g carbohydrates

5 g protein

2 g fat

66 calories

BUTTERSCOTCH PIE

This quick and easy pie is a basic pudding with a crust that cooks in only 5 minutes. The flavor of the filling can be changed simply by exchanging butterscotch flavoring with vanilla, almond or mint.

75 mL	margarine	1/3 cup
250 mL	rolled oats	1 cup
175 mL	crushed walnuts	3/4 cup
500 mL	skim milk	2 cups
25 mL	cornstarch	2 tbsp
1	egg	1
10 mL	butterscotch flavoring	2 tsp
	Sweetener equivalent to	
	50 mL (3 tbsp) sugar	

In a microwave-safe pie plate, melt margarine at High for 30 to 45 seconds. Add rolled oats. Microwave on High for 2 to 3 minutes or until beginning to turn golden brown. Add walnuts. Press mixture onto sides of pie plate and heat at High for 1 minute. Set aside.

In a 1 L (1-quart) measure, microwave milk at High for 4 to 5 minutes or until hot. Stir in cornstarch with a whisk. Microwave at High for 2 to 3 minutes or until mixture begins to thicken. Place egg in a small bowl. Add a small amount of hot milk to egg and stir. Pour egg into milk. Add butterscotch flavoring and sweetener. Pour filling into crust. Chill for 3 to 4 hours before serving.

MAKES	8 servings
EACH SERVING	1/8 wedge

2 FATS AND OILS CHOICES	9 g carbohydrates
1 FRUITS AND VEGETABLES CHOICE	4.4 g protein
1/2 PROTEIN CHOICE	14.8 g fat
	196 calories

CHOCOLATE PIE

175 mL	all-purpose flour	3/4 cup
125 mL	rolled oats	1/2 cup
	Salt to taste	
50 mL	vegetable oil	4 tbsp
40 to 50 mL	ice water	3 to 4 tbsp
1 pkg	plain gelatin	1 pkg
375 mL	skim milk	1-1/2 cups
50 mL	unsweetened cocoa powder	1/4 cup
15 mL	cornstarch	1 tbsp
1	egg, separated	1
	Artificial sweetener equivalent to 125 mL	(1/2 cup) sugar
5 mL	vanilla	1 tsp
50 mL	instant skim milk powder	1/4 cup
50 mL	ice water	1/4 cup

Combine flour, rolled oats and salt in a mixing bowl. Slowly drizzle in oil, mixing with a fork, until mixture resembles fine crumbs. Add ice water a few drops at a time until mixture starts to form a ball. Press into 22 cm (9-in) pie plate. Microwave at High for 4 for 6 minutes, watching carefully to prevent scorching. Allow to cool before filling.

Sprinkle gelatin over 50 mL (1/4 cup) milk to soften. Let stand 5 minutes. In a 2 L (2-quart) measure or bowl, whisk 250 mL (1 cup) milk with cocoa until well mixed. Microwave at Medium Low (50%) for 3 to 5 minutes or until boiling. Reduce power to Low (30%) and microwave for 5 minutes. Combine cornstarch, egg yolk and 50 mL (1/4 cup) milk and stir into cocoa mixture. Microwave at Medium Low (50%) for 1-1/2 to 2 minutes or until mixture thickens. Mix in gelatin and sweetener, stirring until dissolved. Stir in vanilla. Refrigerate until partially set.

Combine egg white, skim milk powder and ice water, and beat until stiff peaks form. Fold into chocolate mixture. Pour into pie crust. Refrigerate 4 hours before serving.

MAKES	8 servings
EACH SERVING	1/8 wedge

1 STARCHY CHOICE	17 g carbohydrates
1/2 MILK CHOICE	6 g protein
1 FATS AND OILS CHOICE	9 g fat
	173 calories

LEMON CHIFFON PIE

50 mL	butter OR margarine	3 tbsp
175 mL	graham wafer crumbs	3/4 cup
1 mL	cinnamon	1/4 tsp
1 mL	nutmeg	1/4 tsp
0.5 mL	allspice	1/8 tsp
1 pkg	plain gelatin	1 pkg
125 mL	water	1/2 cup
2	eggs, separated	2
50 mL	sugar	3 tbsp
2 mL	grated lemon peel	1/2 tsp
0.5 mL	salt	1/8 tsp
50 mL	lemon juice	1/4 cup
	Artificial sweetener equivalent to 125 mL (1/2 cup) sugar	
75 mL	powdered skim milk	1/3 cup
75 mL	ice water	1/3 cup
15 mL	lemon juice	1 tbsp

Melt butter or margarine in a pie plate at High for 30 to 45 seconds. Combine graham wafer crumbs, cinnamon, nutmeg and allspice. Add to pie plate and combine well with a fork. Spread evenly over bottom of pie plate. Microwave at High for 3 to 5 minutes, watching carefully to prevent scorching. Allow to cool before filling.

In a large measure, sprinkle gelatin on 125 mL (1/2 cup) water. Allow to soften. In a separate bowl, combine egg yolks, sugar, lemon peel, salt and 50 mL (1/4 cup) lemon juice. Microwave at Medium (70%) for 5 to 8 minutes until mixture comes to a boil, stirring every 2 minutes. Add gelatin and sweetener and mix well. Refrigerate until slightly thickened.

Beat egg whites, powdered milk, ice water and 15 mL (1 tbsp) lemon juice until stiff. Carefully fold gelatin mixture into egg whites. Pour into crust. Refrigerate for 2 hours before serving.

MAKES	8 servings
EACH SERVING	1/8 wedge

1 STARCHY CHOICE	15 g carbohydrates
1 FATS AND OILS CHOICE	4 g protein
	5 g fat
	115 calories

PUMPKIN LIGHT PIE

Freeze any leftovers for a diabetic treat some other time.

50 mL	butter OR margarine	3 tbsp
175 mL	graham wafer crumbs	3/4 cup
15 mL	plain gelatin	1 tbsp
125 mL	cold water	1/2 cup
3	eggs, separated	3
125 mL	skim milk	1/2 cup
1	can (306 mL/1-1/4 cups) pumpkin	1
2 mL	salt	1/2 tsp
1 mL	nutmeg	1/4 tsp
3 mL	cinnamon	3/4 tsp
2 mL	ginger	1/2 tsp
2 mL	allspice	1/2 tsp
	Artificial sweetener equivalent to 125 mL (1/2 cup) sugar	
25 mL	sugar	2 tbsp

Melt butter or margarine in a 1 L (9-in) pie plate at High for 30 to 40 seconds. Add graham wafer crumbs to pie plate and combine well with a fork. Spread evenly over bottom of pie plate. Microwave at High for 3 to 5 minutes, watching carefully to prevent scorching. Allow to cool before filling.

Dissolve gelatin in cold water and set aside. Beat egg yolks in a 2 L (2-quart) measure or mixing bowl. Stir in milk, pumpkin, salt and spices. Mix well. Microwave at Medium Low (50%) for 3 to 4 minutes until thick and smooth, stirring 2 to 3 times. If more cooking time is needed to thicken, microwave at Medium Low (50%) for 30-second intervals until thick and smooth, stirring after each interval. Add gelatin and sweetener. Stir until completely dissolved. Refrigerate until the thickness of unbeaten egg whites.

Beat egg whites until soft peaks form. Gradually add sugar and continue beating until stiff and shiny. Fold into pumpkin mixture, being careful to combine thoroughly. Pour into prepared pie shell. Chill overnight.

MAKES	8 servings
EACH SERVING	1/8 wedge

. . . .

1 STARCHY CHOICE	16 g carbohydrates
1 PROTEIN CHOICE	5 g protein
1 FATS AND OILS CHOICE	8 g fat
	168 calories

WINTER FRUIT PUDDING

This delicious pudding is made from apples and dried fruits, making it very convenient to prepare from stock in the cupboards. The old-fashioned pudding lends itself to a topping of milk or cream.

. . . .

125 mL	apple slices	1/2 cup
125 mL	dried prunes	1/2 cup
50 mL	dried apricots	1/4 cup
	Juice of 1 orange	
250 mL	whole-wheat flour	1 cup
5 mL	cinnamon	1/2 tsp
75 mL	skim milk	1/3 cup

. . . .

Combine fruits with orange juice. Stir and cover. Microwave at High for 2 minutes or until juice boils. Let stand to rehydrate fruit for 5 minutes. In a 1 L (1-quart) measure, combine flour, cinnamon and milk. Press onto sides of measure and microwave at Medium (70%) for 2 to 3 minutes or until dry to the touch. Fill with fruit mixture. Allow 5 minutes aftercooking time. Turn out of measure to serve.

. . . .

| MAKES | 6 servings |
| EACH SERVING | 100 mL (1/3 cup plus 2 tbsp) |

. . . .

1 STARCHY CHOICE	27 g carbohydrates
1 FRUITS AND VEGETABLES CHOICE	3 g protein
	121 calories

VANILLA PUDDING

This wonderful basic pudding requires only 6 to 7 minutes to cook. Allow for chilling time when you plan to use this recipe for dinner.

500 mL	skim milk	2 cups
25 mL	cornstarch	2 tbsp
1	egg	1
10 mL	vanilla	2 tsp
	Sweetener equivalent to	
	25 mL (2 tbsp) sugar	

In a 1 L (1-quart) measure, microwave milk at High for 4 to 5 minutes or until hot. Whisk in cornstarch. Microwave at High for 2 to 3 minutes or until mixture begins to thicken. Place egg in a small bowl. Pour a small amount of hot milk onto egg. Stir. Pour egg into milk. Add vanilla and sweetener. Chill thoroughly before serving.

MAKES	4 servings
EACH SERVING	125 mL (1/2 cup)

1 MILK CHOICE	6 g carbohydrates
	4.5 g protein
	1.2 g fat
	53 calories

APPLE JELLY

Jelly is the perfect spread for toast, breads and cakes. This one takes only 3 minutes to cook, and stores well in the refrigerator for up to two weeks.

250 mL	apple juice	1 cup
15 mL	lemon juice	1 tbsp
50 mL	liquid pectin	1/4 cup
	Sweetener equivalent to	
	25 mL (2 tbsp) sugar	

In a 500 mL (2-cup) measure, combine apple juice and lemon juice. Microwave at High for 2-1/2 to 3 minutes or until boiling. Stir in pectin and sweetener. Pour jelly into sterilized jar and store in refrigerator.

....

MAKES   325 mL (1-1/3 cups)
EACH SERVING   15 mL (1 tbsp)

....

1/2 EXTRA CHOICE   1.3 g carbohydrates

                                                              5 calories

STRAWBERRY JAM

Made with fresh or frozen strawberries, this jam is quick and tasty. Store in the refrigerator for up to two weeks, or in the freezer. You certainly can't beat the flavor and calorie count!

....

500 mL	fresh or frozen strawberries	2 cups
1/2 box	powdered pectin	1/2 box
125 mL	water	1/2 cup
	Sweetener equivalent to	
	50 mL (1/4 cup) sugar	

....

In a 1 L (1-quart) casserole, heat strawberries at High for 5 to 6 minutes or until boiling in own juice. Add pectin and water. Microwave at High for 1 minute. Stir. Add sweetener. Pour into sterilized jar and store in refrigerator.

....

MAKES   625 mL (2-1/2 cups)
EACH SERVING   15 mL (1 tbsp)

....

1 EXTRA CHOICE   .6 g carbohydrates

                                                        3 calories

RECIPES ADAPTED FROM CHOICE COOKING, NC PRESS

Clear Mushroom Soup
Minestrone Soup
Basic White Sauce
Mushroom Gravy
Spaghetti Sauce
Salisbury Steak
Swiss Mocha Delight
Cream of Celery Soup
Fat-Free No-Lump Gravy
Prairie Pot Roast
Chicken Paprika
Italian Chicken
Creamy Cheese and Macaroni

Turkey Tetrazzini
Microwaved Burger Pizza
Shepherd's Pie
Bran Muffins
Date-Nut Bran Muffins
Shortbread
Microwaved Chocolate Chip
  Cookies
Easy Stew
Oatmeal Pie Crust
Graham Cracker Pie Crust
Chocolate Delight
Chocolate Pie

RECIPES BY CHOICE GROUP

STARCHY CHOICES RECIPES

INDEX